Disaster Preparedness Guide
Mitigation, Rescue and Coping Skills

FRED MAJIWA

Disaster Preparedness Guide: Mitigation, Rescue and Coping Skills

Authored by: Fred Majiwa

Revised Edition February 2018

Published by:
CreateSpace, a Subsidiary of Amazon
4900 LaCross Road
North Charleston, South Carolina 29406
USA

www.createspace.com

Disclaimer:
The author of this guidebook is not a physician, and enclosed suggestions should not replace advice of a trained Medical Practitioner. All the content here is for informational purpose only, and neither the author nor publisher can accept injury, loss or damage arising from this information. During a time of disasters, people should heed the advice of disaster officials over the information contained in this book.

Email: fredmajiwa@gmail.com
Phone: +254 780 188555

ISBN-13: 978-1533494986
ISBN-10: 1533494983

ISBN 978-1-5334-9498-6

US$15.00

51500>

9 781533 494986

IN MEMORIAM

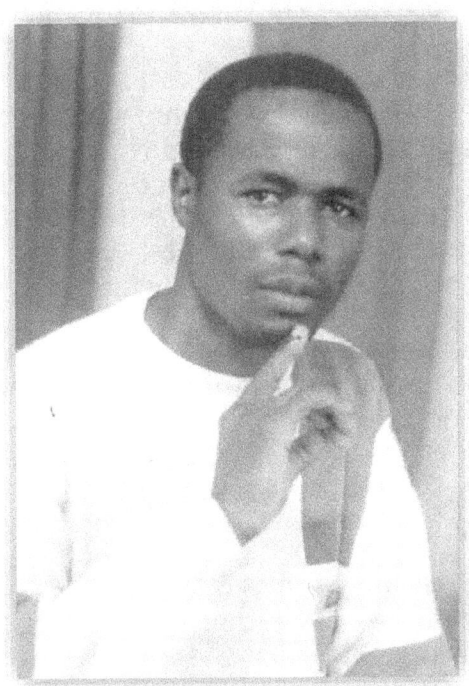

Sam Majiwa died in a tragic road accident on Jogoo Road in Nairobi on 17th December 2005. His body was discovered at the City Mortuary after 23 days, when some parts had started decomposing.

This horrific incident cut short his ambition of becoming a Civil Engineer when he was in his final year of studies at the University of Nairobi.

The death of Sam was heartbreaking, especially to the family and close friends, just like those of nearly 3,000 people crashed to death on Kenyan roads every year.

In memoriam, his younger brother Fred Majiwa authored this handbook to help thousands cut down road carnage and other fatal disasters that dominate Kenya's profile.

FOREWORD

Kenya has experienced a worrying trend of fatal disasters in the recent past, leaving a trail of death and destruction.

Among the cases that stirred the nation's conscience was the terror attacks at Westgate Mall and Garissa University, in which more than 200 people were massacred.

Another calamity that Kenyans have to contend with is the rising cases of fatal fire disasters, especially in urban slums, boarding schools, and on the road by fuel tankers.

The country also experiences severe droughts and serious incidents of floods. Other calamities are collapsing buildings, rampant road crashes, and violent crimes.

Response to these disasters is often inadequate and characterized by failure to act on early warnings.

As a result, people often find it easy to point accusing finger to the ill-preparedness of authorities in dealing with the calamities. But one thing that the whole world agrees is that safety begins with everyone.

As authorities are trying to put their acts together, each person can play a vital role in improving their personal preparedness to deal with common emergencies around them.

It is in the realization of this need for personal preparation that this *Disaster Preparedness Guide* was authored by Fred Majiwa - a disaster expert with many years of experience as a senior manager at the St John Ambulance.

In a language that's easy for anyone to get through, the book helps people to learn how to deal with nearly all disasters in the country.

It also includes comprehensive first aid and counselling guidelines, focusing on prevention, than merely responding to emergencies after they occur.

Contents

PART I: DISASTER PREPAREDNESS

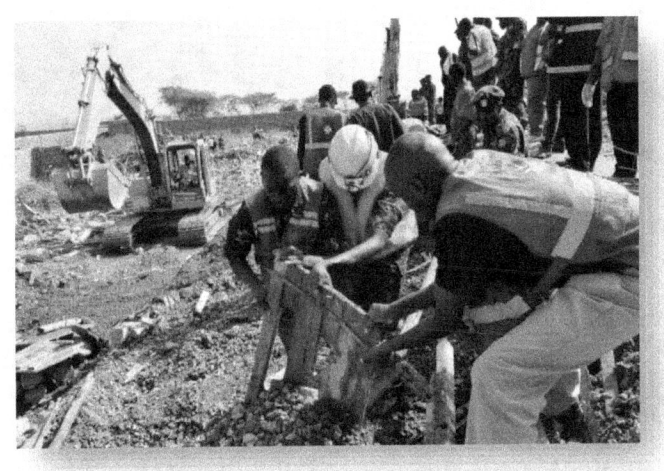

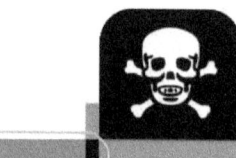

KENYA'S DISASTER PROFILE

Kenya is among the low-income nations, which are more vulnerable to disasters, and the need for preparedness cannot be overemphasized.

Communities are predisposed to calamities by a combination of factors such as poverty, drought, settlement in areas prone to perennial flooding or even living in poorly constructed buildings.

In the recent past these hazards have increased in number, frequency and complexity.

The level of destruction has also become more severe, with more deaths of people and animals, loss of livelihoods, destruction of infrastructure among other effects resulting in losses of varying magnitudes.

Response to disasters is often inadequate and characterized by failure to act on early warnings and safety precautions.

For instance, when people get serious El Niño warnings for months, the only preparations you can notably see are buying of umbrellas on the streets and at local supermarkets, instead of reinforcing weak walls and unblocking of household drainage systems.

> "when people get serious El Niño warnings for months, the only preparations you can notably see are buying of umbrellas at local supermarkets"

People often find it easy to point accusing finger to the ill-preparedness of the authorities in dealing with calamities.

But one thing that the whole world agrees is that safety begins with everyone.

As authorities are trying to put their acts together, each person can play a vital role in improving their personal preparedness to deal with common emergencies around them.

The country's profile is dominated by manmade disasters including terror attacks, fire outbreaks, road carnage, collapsing buildings, violent crimes, conflicts and disease outbreaks.

Luckily, there's no significant natural disasters other than weather-related calamities such as drought, floods and landslides.

This disaster profile makes Kenya unique from other parts of the world which are predominantly affected by natural hazards, including tornadoes, tsunami, earthquakes, and heatwaves.

Some of the specific tragedies have been highlighted in the following section:

Terror attacks

The threat of terrorism remains the most scary disaster risk in Kenya.

The country has been a fertile ground for series of severe terror attacks, often carried out in populous cities such as Nairobi as well as coastal and northern counties.

> "Following these spate of attacks, many people now live in fear, spread over further promised retaliations"

August 7, 2008 bombing of the US embassy in Nairobi remains the deadliest in Kenya's history. 213 people were killed, while at least 4,000 more were wounded.

In April 2015, students at Garissa University College were attacked by Al Shabaab gunmen. At least 148 were massacred, in what was described as the second worst terrorist attack in the country.

In another horrific attack, the group killed 67 people during a four-day siege at Westgate shopping mall in the capital, Nairobi, in September 2013.

Following these spate of attacks, many people now live in fear, spread over further promised retaliations.

Violent crimes

Another disaster that Kenyans have to contend with, especially those in urban areas, is greater level of violent crime, which gets dangerous during night hours.

For instance, Nairobi has struggled with rising crime, earning a nickname "Nairobbery".

Some of the most dangerous crooks responsible for violent crimes such as carjacking, robberies, and raping are local gangs formed by teenagers in informal settlements.

Ethnic violence also occur frequently, due to unresolved border conflicts, cattle rustling, competition over land and water resources, and political conflict.

These conflicts lead to exoduses of ethnic minority communities with roots in other geographical areas.

The worst crisis to hit Kenya was in December 2007. About 1,500 people were killed and 600,000 displaced after the disputed presidential election.

Fire Outbreaks

Fire is another frequent disaster. A week barely passes before a fire incident is reported, mostly in congested slums and boarding schools.

The informal settlements have become a death trap for many people, some of whom have died in mysterious fire disasters.

The most horrible was the Sinai fire tragedy in September 2011, where as many as 120 people were burnt beyond recognition when a pipeline burst into flames as slum dwellers were siphoning fuel from it.

In slums, fire engines are in many occasions reduced to mere spectators, extinguishing flames at the periphery, as there is no access roads and every square inch of land is occupied.

This worrying trend of fatal fire disasters is also creeping into boarding schools.

Among the cases that stirred the nation's conscience was the 2017 Moi Girls High school fire, where nine students died.

In 2001, 68 boys were burnt to death in Kyanguli Secondary School fire in Machakos. In the same year, in Bombolulu Girls at the Coast, 58 children died in a dormitory fire.

More than 120 schools were burnt in a wave of arson attacks in 2016, leading to student deaths, loss of property worth millions and disruption of learning.

Floods and Flash Floods

The country has also experienced serious incidents of floods and flash floods in different parts of the country.

During these flooding, there are incidences of terrible traffic jams, and commuters spending nights in their cars due to impassable roads.

Lives are lost by drowning, electrocution, and landslide. Homes are also marooned, and poorly built structures collapse.

But more upsetting is that, most fatalities occur because people underestimate the strength of moving water and ignore safety advices with fatal consequences.

> "most fatalities occur because people underestimate the strength of moving water"

For instance, motorists are swept while attempting to cross swollen rivers that overflow over bridges, instead of being patient for water levels to subside.

Drought

Compared to other extreme events, drought tends to be the largest and most costly natural disaster in the country, with the highest potential damage to agriculture, energy and water sectors.

As result of perennial droughts, about two million people are permanently in need of food aid, especially in arid and semi-arid areas which occupy 80 percent of Kenya. These dry areas are home to approximately 30 percent (12 million) of Kenya's people and 50 percent of its livestock.

In recent years, the country has experienced severe droughts. In 2000, at least 4 million people were in need of food aid after Kenya was hit by its worst drought in 37 years.

Early 2017, the government declared drought affecting 23 arid and semi-arid counties a national disaster.

Most of those at risk are small-scale herders in arid and semi-arid lands, where livestock rearing account for as much as 90 percent of employment and family income.

In urban areas, however, where thousands have flocked in search of hard-to-come by jobs, hunger ravages families not because there is no food to buy, but people cannot afford.

Prices of most basic foods that commonly include sukuma wiki, rice, and maize flour rise due to prevailing drought conditions, making them inaccessible.

Collapsing Buildings

The cases of structural failures and consequent collapse of buildings, more specifically in urban areas, has also reached an alarming state in the past few years.

In May 2016, a seven-storey building which was dangerously constructed on the riparian area collapsed, killing 51 people in Huruma Estate, Nairobi.

Earlier in 2014, a five-storey building that was partly occupied and still under construction collapsed in Kaloleni. Seven people died in the incident. Three weeks later, another building collapsed in Huruma, killing five people.

In 2015, seventeen buildings collapsed, including a case in Roysambu along Thika Road where seven people died.

These cases exemplifies the many incidences that tenants have been subjected to dangerous occupancy, resulting into loss of lives and property worth millions of shillings.

A number of reasons have been cited to explain why these buildings collapse, including poor-workmanship, use of substandard materials and multitude of other reasons.

Road Carnage

Road accident is fast becoming an almost weekly ritual, especially at the notorious blackspots along the northern corridor and other major highways.

One of the worst incidences in recent history is the alarming death of at least 43 people in a road crash at Laini, Naivasha along Nairobi-Nakuru highway in December 2016, which gripped many with sorrow, fury and outrage.

Many lives were needlessly lost, just like those of nearly 3,000 people killed in road crash each and every year in Kenya.

These deaths uphold a report released in 2015 by the World Health Organization (WHO), that rank roads in Kenya among some of the world's dangerous highways.

Some of the deadly behaviors to blame for the road toll include drunken driving, speeding and dangerous overtaking.

Overlapping matatus and boda-boda operators, who violate traffic regulations also contribute substantially to road deaths.

Matatus, which are the commonly used means of public transport, are driven at breakneck speed, overlap, cut into queues, hoot incessantly, play loud music and obstruct other motorists. The not-so-lucky passengers also get assaulted.

These uncourteous manners are not limited to public transport. Indeed, some of the bad practice has rubbed off on private motorists and many view each other with disgust.

But more inexcusable is that, more than half of all the road deaths are as a result of mishandling by responders who lack basic knowledge on first aid.

Disease Outbreaks

Rise in disease outbreaks such as Cholera has also recently affected many parts of the country, with confirmed fatal cases and acute dehydration.

Lack of toilets and poor sanitation have been blamed for increasing cases of disease outbreaks.

Alcohol Poisoning

Consumption of illicit brews is also so prevalent to an extent consumers literally live in the dens of the deadly concoctions, oblivious of its fatal consequences.

Recently, the media has been awash with reports of unfortunate deaths and blindness arising from consumption of illicit brews.

Cases of drink-spiking in pubs is also increasingly worrying, particularly male revelers who are the main targets.

Chemical spillage

To end the list of disasters is chemical spillage, which has in the past affected *Juakali* areas, where artisans handling scrap metals and waste containers are exposed to toxic gases and other chemicals.

But more intolerable is that populations are still living on top of the petroleum pipeline passing through Sinai area in Nairobi, despite the fact that more than 120 people lost their lives on the same spot when underground oil tunnel exploded.

Some incidents of spillage are also witnessed during storage and transportation of fuels and other hazardous materials by tankers. These mostly occurs near black spot areas along the northern corridor.

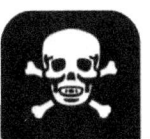

1.1 Need for Personal Preparedness

When Al-Shabaab gunmen opened fire on shoppers at the Westgate Mall, killing 67 people and wounding over 200 others, disaster rescue teams responded to the incident.

However, before the teams arrived, there were ordinary civilians helping victims run for cover, evacuating the wounded and giving basic first aid.

They never knew an emergency situation will occur, and their help will be needed. Instantly, they transitioned from simple bystanders to lifesavers.

The Westgate tragedy, along with other mass casualty incidents, drives home the need for everyone, not just first responders, to have the knowledge to deal with calamities and provide immediate care prior to the arrival of advanced help.

Being prepared helps people to cope with the aftermath of a disaster and be an asset to community in a serious emergency.

A great first step towards being prepared is to identify the potential dangers that may exist in the surrounding and find ways of mitigating their impacts.

For instance, if you live in an area that is prone to flooding, it is important to take necessary steps like moving to safer grounds, reinforcing weak walls or unblocking drainage systems to protect your home from flooding.

Attending first aid or disaster preparedness course and having a plan of action on how to deal with specific types of emergency situations can also go a long way towards reducing the fear and anxiety that can arise from the unknown.

Subsequently, stock a first aid kit, fire extinguisher and other survival items like water purifiers and flashlight to ensure you have all of the necessary items for basic survival. Other items to consider stocking in the same place are backup means of charging cellphones and emergency hotlines for police, fire and ambulance services.

It is also crucial to check on your emergency kits approximately every six months for expired medications and other outdated requiring replacements.

Financial plan is equally essential in your disaster preparedness. Try to have five-days' worth of cash to use in the event you can't get to your local bank or ATMs are not available. Online banking is one of the ways to manage your finances during unsettled times.

Finally, consider risk insurance for disasters that can inflict personal losses you cannot recover from easily, to increases the chances of returning to normalcy faster.

1.2 Phases of Disaster Management

D isaster preparedness is just one phase in disaster management cycle. The other phases include: prevention, response, and recovery as illustrated in the figure below:

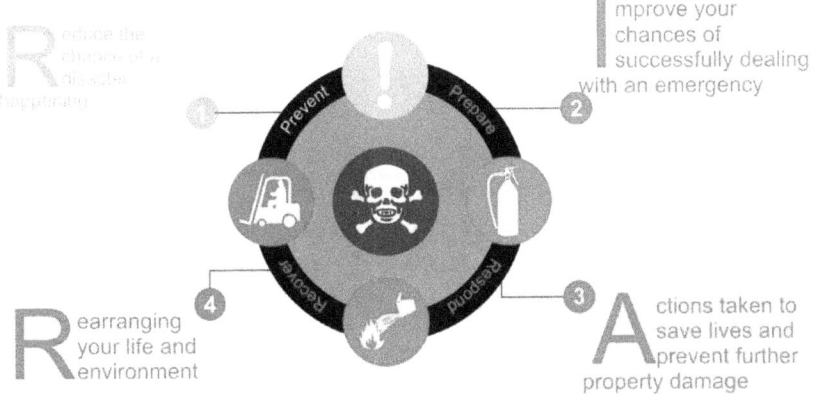

Figure 1: Phases of Disaster Management

Phase 1: Prevention and Mitigation

This phase includes any activity that prevent and reduce the chance of a disaster happening, or reduce the damaging effects of unavoidable emergencies.

For example, to mitigate fire in your home, follow safety standards in selecting wiring and appliances.

But an accident involving fire could still happen even with the best preparedness. Therefore, you need to buy a fire insurance to protect yourself from the costly burden of rebuilding after fire incident.

Phase 2: Preparedness

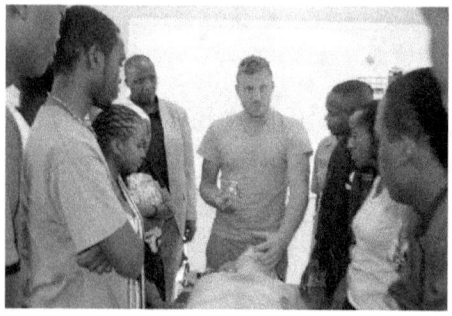

Figure 2: Basic Life Support Training

This phase includes developing contingency plans, learning lifesaving skills, and other actions that will improve your chances of successfully dealing with an emergency.

For instance, posting emergency telephone numbers, holding disaster drills, and installing smoke detectors are all preparedness measures.

You should also consider setting up an emergency fund and preparing a disaster kit with essential supplies.

Phase 3:Response

Response to a disaster event must be swift and effective to combat the disaster, to assist those affected by it, and to make the area safe.

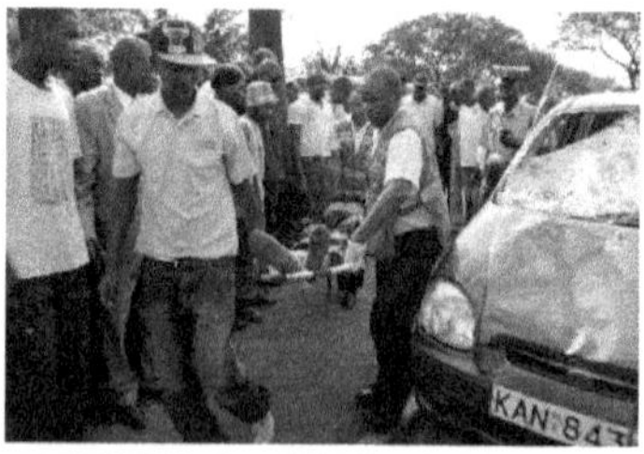

It includes actions taken to save lives and prevent further property damage. Your well-being depend on your preparedness to respond to a crisis.

Figure 3: Emergency Medics respond to a road crash incident

This phase includes actions taken to return to normalcy or safer situation following an emergency.

Once the immediate danger is over, your continued well-being depends on your ability to cope with rearranging your life and environment.

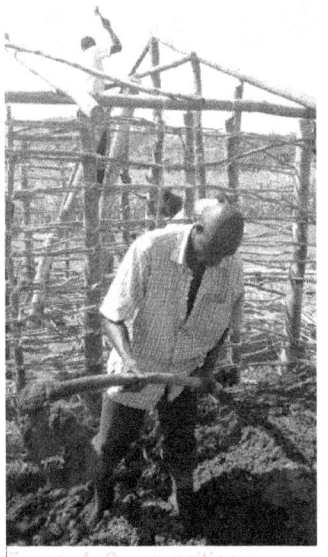

You must take care of yourself to prevent stress-related illnesses and excessive financial burdens.

During recovery, you should also consider things to do that would lessen (mitigate) the effects of future disasters.

Figure 4: Communities participating in reconstruction of their member's house

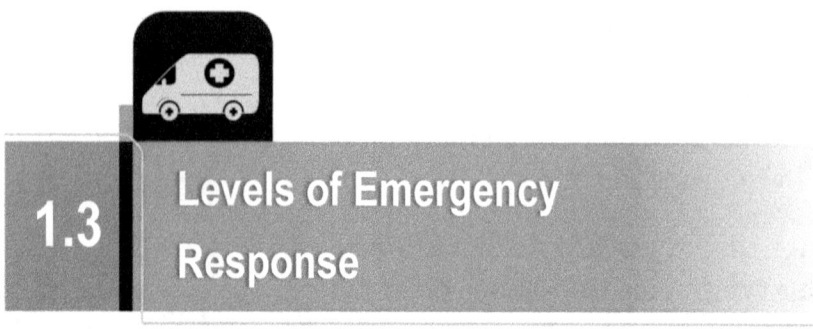

1.3 Levels of Emergency Response

It is much better to take actions to stay safe by preventing disaster risks, or at the very least, mitigate their impacts on livelihoods and property, than just responding to them.

However, disasters may still occur even with the best level of prevention and mitigation.

When these disasters occur, many people find it easy to blame authorities for not doing enough to prepare and respond to the dangers facing civilians.

However, the reality is that proper response is best achieved when you, your local community and the government are all prepared to respond, as highlighted in the three levels below:

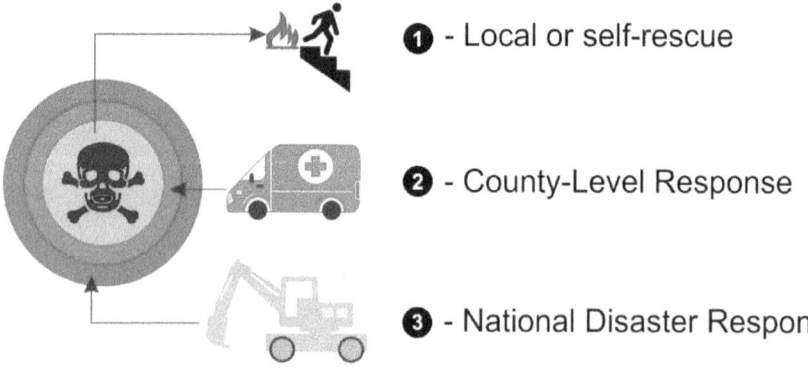

❶ - Local or self-rescue

❷ - County-Level Response

❸ - National Disaster Response

Figure 5: Levels of emergency response

Self or Local Rescue

Self or local rescue is the first and most important level of response.

During this stage, the locals try to use available resources within their level of knowledge to survive the emergency.

For instance, during fire or terrorism incident, it is important that the locals know how to respond, as these disasters have a tendency of escalating fast before rescue teams arrive at scene.

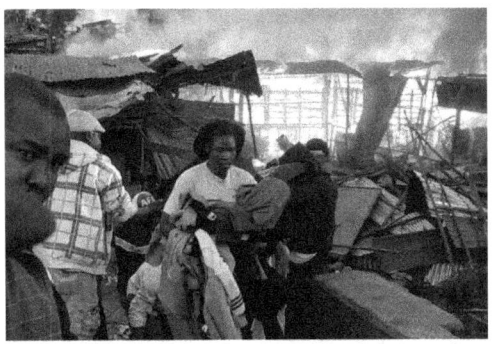

Figure 6: Slum residents salvage property after a fire outbreak

Some people prepare and survive by taking control of the situation, while others panic as they wait for help from authorities, worsening their chances of survival.

The authorities may provide assistance during disasters, but that may take several hours if not days in particular situations.

This is why everyone needs to take initiative to prepare for and respond to emergencies that may occur in their locality, and be ready to be self-sufficient after an incident, until external assistance from authorities arrive.

Some of the recommended ways of becoming disaster ready at local level are:

- ➲ Assess the possible dangers in the surrounding.

- ➲ Take training in first aid and disaster preparedness.

- Install a first aid kit, smoke detector and fire extinguisher.

- Create a simple emergency plan and rehearse it.

- Take disaster alerts seriously and learn the evacuation routes.

- Volunteer with disaster agencies to help others.

- Report suspicious activities, especially terror suspects.

County Level Response

The second level of emergency response is the county response teams, including private and non-governmental agencies.

The specific responsibilities of county authorities in emergency management include:

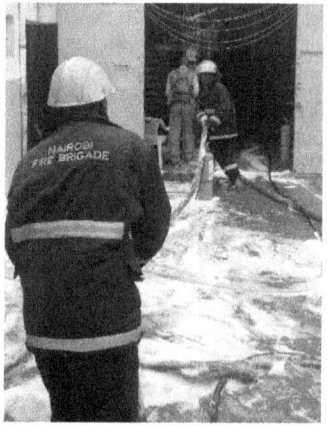

Figure 7: County fire officials putting out an inferno in an industrial godown in Nairobi

- Identifying hazards and assessing their potential risk to local communities.

- Providing ambulances and firefighting services.

- Improving coordination and cooperation with other governmental and non-governmental agencies.

- Establishing mitigation measures such as building codes, or land-use management programs.

- Developing and coordinating contingency plans.

- Establishing early-warning systems.

- Stocking disaster supplies and equipment.

- Training the public and emergency personnel.

National Disaster Response

If damages are so extensive that the combined local and county resources are not sufficient, there is need for assistance from the national disaster agencies.

At the moment, there are several national agencies involved at this level, including the National Disaster Operation Center, Military Disaster Response Unit, Disaster Management Unit of the National Police Service, and non-governmental agencies.

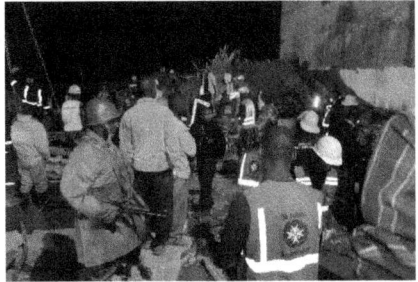

Figure 8: National Response Teams at a site of a collapsed building in Mlolongo, Machakos County

It would be ideal if a national disaster management authority is established, so that some of its roles would include:

- Development and review of national policies, strategies and plans for disaster reduction.

- Formulation of standards and licensing of emergency organizations.

- Coordination of national disaster response and recovery activities.

- Mobilization of resources and financial assistance to counties and local non-governmental agencies.

- Conducting of research and training programs on first aid and disaster risk management.

Declaration of National Disaster

If the magnitude of the disaster overwhelms the national capacity, then the president may declare a national disaster and seek international support.

The United Nations or African Union may also veto a decision to send peacekeeping units to coordinate humanitarian activities in well-deserving cases such as political crisis where the head of state is implicated.

Role of voluntary organizations

Some of the most important voluntary organizations in terms of disasters is the St John Ambulance and Red Cross.

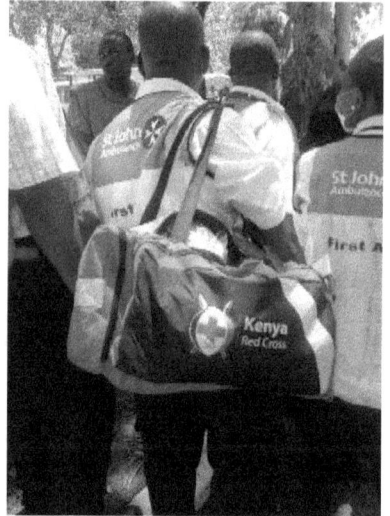

They provide individuals and families with first aid, medicines, food, shelter, clothing, bedding, counselling and other services.

Voluntary organizations also conduct fund-raising drives to provide financial assistance to disaster victims.

Disaster Management at Workplace

Protecting the lives and improving wellbeing of workers has positive ramifications on a firm's productivity.

Additionally, employment and labor laws also requires employers to:

- ⮑ Employ an officer in charge of safety, if having more than 25 employees.

- Create an occupational safety committee to oversee safety management issues.

- Assess occupational hazards and mitigate impacts.

- Install adequately stocked first aid kits and firefighting equipment.

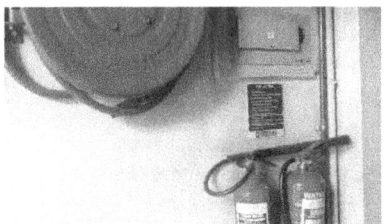

- Install proper signage e.g. fire exit, assembly, fire management steps.

Figure 9: Firefighting equipment at workplace

- Create a first aid room and employ a nurse if having more than 500 workers.

- Conduct firefighting and first aid training to at least two in every 25 workers per shift.

- Develop contingency or disaster response plans.

- Conduct drills to test contingency plans and evacuation procedures.

- Contract and develop liaison with an ambulance service and firefighting agency.

1.4 | Disaster Impact Assessment

Disasters are characterized by overwhelming needs and competing priorities. Given this nature, damage assessment is crucial to help convey the 'situation on the ground' to effectively mobilize resources.

Assessment also identifies critical needs and prescribe the priorities for response and recovery activities. Assessment can be rapid or comprehensive.

Rapid Assessment

Rapid or initial assessment comprise of both situation assessments and needs analyses in the early disaster stage.

The assessment helps to determine the disaster magnitude, its impact and immediate needs for relief assistance.

The following checklist helps in conducting rapid assessment:
- ➲ *General situation*
    - ☐ Type of crisis, date, time, and location of crisis
    - ☐ Most needed items and accessibility of the disaster site
- ➲ *Population*
    - ☐ Number of fatalities, injuries, and missing people
    - ☐ Number of kids, disabled, elderlies, pregnant women
    - ☐ Displaced people in camps or host families
    - ☐ Poverty level and economic activity

Health Situation
- [ ] Available ambulances and health facilities
- [ ] Approximate hospital bed capacities
- [ ] Hospitalized patients and main injuries causes
- [ ] Body management

Water and Sanitation
- [ ] Disruption of water supply and sewer systems
- [ ] Households without water supply
- [ ] Alternative source of water
- [ ] Alternative latrine available
- [ ] Contamination of hydro, air, and ground
- [ ] Risks of disease outbreaks

Food and Nutrition
- [ ] Loss of crops and livestock
- [ ] Effect on harvest and future needs for food
- [ ] Capacity to buy or access food
- [ ] Main food and nutrition needs

Shelter and Nonfood Items
- [ ] Ongoing shelter arrangements (churches, schools)
- [ ] Security in the shelters
- [ ] Lighting, housing and nonfood items e.g. blanket

Livelihood (early recovery)
- [ ] Affected economic activities
- [ ] Availability of markets and effect on commodity prices
- [ ] Available land for relocation

Protection
- [ ] Risk of violent attacks
- [ ] Children separated from their family

- [ ] Reports of mistreatment or sexual abuse
- [ ] Psychosocial support and rights protection agencies
- [ ] Main protection needs and barriers

➲ *Coordination*
- [ ] Lead agency and other active response agencies
- [ ] Ongoing rescue activities and main coordination needs
- [ ] Cellular networks available

➲ *Education*
- [ ] Affected schools
- [ ] Number of students in disaster zone
- [ ] Estimated loss in school property
- [ ] Main education needs

Comprehensive Assessment

An in-depth assessment usually starts after the initial assessments. It covers critical areas to be addressed for medium-and long-term relief and reconstruction assistance.

This assessment is best completed by team of experts, and begin as rapid or initial assessments are coming to an end. There may even be some overlap.

Reports

The reports derived from the rapid assessment are the Situation Reports (SitReps) and the Flash Appeal (if necessary). The following formats may be used:

Situation Reports

- Date/Time.
- Situation: Disaster type, affected area, impact, projection of threats.
- Internal response: Local, county and national disaster authorities, coordination, limitations.
- Assistance for priority needs.
- Logistics and channels for contributions.

Flash Appeal

- Executive Summary: The crisis, priority needs, required amount of financial resources, time of implementation of the flash appeal resources.
- Context and humanitarian consequences: Ongoing operations, most affected population, immediate needs, and priorities.

Response Plan: Included for each aspect such as search and rescue, medical, psychosocial support, and tracing.

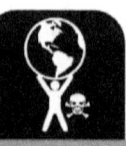

1.5 | Global Perspectives in Disaster Risk Reduction

Disaster risk reduction policies and strategies around the globe are guided by the international frameworks, currently Sendai Framework 2015-2030 which was developed after ratification of Hyogo Framework 2005-2015.

The new framework placed strong emphasis on disaster risk management as opposed to disaster management. Significance was also laid on the preventing new risk while reducing existing ones and strengthening resilience.

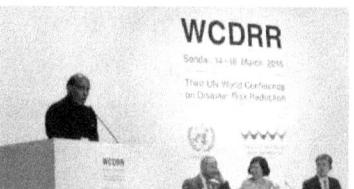

Figure 10: World Conference on Disaster Risk Reduction ongoing at Sendai, Japan

The scope of disaster risk reduction was also broadened significantly to focus on environmental, technological and biological hazards in addition to natural and man-made disaster risks.

The Sendai Framework articulated the following four priority areas:

Pillar 1: Understanding Disaster Risk

The framework buoys up the use of suitable technology to put in place a database to collect disaster data for evaluation, dissemination, training, research, awareness and campaigns.

Pillar 2: Strengthening governance

Institutionalizing disaster management, by putting in place a disaster management authority, is very key in championing the implementation of strategies and taking responsibility for the outcomes.

Other areas encouraged under this pillar include tax relief for promotion of disaster preparedness, capacity building of responders, and coordination forums at local, county, and national levels.

Pillar 3: Investing in disaster risk reduction

To fulfill this priority, authorities are urged to allocate resources in their budgets, insure some disasters, and strengthen enforcement of safety laws.

Other aspects include investing in workplace resilience, livelihood enhancement, environmental management, poverty eradication, and food security.

Pillar 4: Enhancing disaster preparedness

This priority is fulfilled by putting in place early warning systems, disaster response equipment, emergency fund, relief stockpiling, training of first responders, public awareness, urban planning and relocation of risky habitats.

Contingency plans also need to be drafted and subjected to mock drills to confirm readiness and ability.

Hefty fines for failure to help an emergency victim

Unlike back in the days before Kenyans fell in love with litigation, people used to help one another, without worrying about possible consequences if something went wrong.

For instance, neighbors would wake up in the middle of the night to help whenever someone screamed for help.

But this days, there is a lot in the media about people being sued, until others can be afraid to act, even to help one another, for fear of being sued if something goes wrong.

In such emergency or disaster circumstance, one of the most common questions people ask before giving help is "will I get sued if I help a casualty then she succumbs to her injuries?"

This is a reasonable question given the increasingly litigious situation in the country, with lawsuits being very common.

However, there is no chance of being found legally liable, If you do everything in the best interest of the victim or as trained, even if the victim does not recover.

The most important thing to remember is that, to date, no one in Kenya has ever been sued for administering life-saving help to a disaster victim.

Although legal problems seldom arises in disaster situations, certain legal concepts highlighted below are important to protect yourself from litigations when giving help at incidents:

Scope of practice

First, always act only within the scope of what you are trained or instructed by a qualified expert. Acting outside your scope, such as trying to do something you heard and have not been trained to do so, may make you legally liable for the results of your action.

Consent

Secondly, seek the victim's consent before giving help. Touching another person without consent may be misconstrued as sexual assault or battery, which is a criminal offence.

However, if the victim is unconscious or parent cannot be reached quickly for consent, then you have an implied consent to offer help.

Abandonment

Subsequently, do not abandon a victim. Keep giving help until someone with advanced skills takeover. If you leave a victim and the condition worsens, this is called abandonment, except if you do so due to exhaustion.

Documentations

It would be advisable to make a diary note of assistance given to a victim. Records should be kept fairly simple and clear, listing an accurate and factual account of your observations only, and not any professional conclusions.

Duty to Act

Finally, the laws impose legal obligation on medics to provide emergency medical treatment to a victim where possible, regardless of the ability to pay.

Professionals like doctors, paramedics or firefighters with a job requirement to offer medical care or disaster rescue have a duty to act, including times when they are off duty, and may be held liable for failing to act or acting inappropriately.

This is highlighted in Article 43(2) of the Constitution as well as Section 7(1) of the Health Act 2017, which states that "a person shall not be denied emergency medical treatment."

Hefty fines for failure to help an emergency victim

Under the Act, institutions may be slammed with hefty fine of up to three million shillings for not giving emergency help to victims. Practitioner's license may also be revoked for not responding to emergency call.

Such medical help entails pre-hospital care, stabilizing of the victims, or arranging for referral to advanced hospital, but may not include admission into the hospital wards.

Parents are also required to provide medical treatment and adequate care to their children. This is under the laws against child abuse and neglect.

On the other hand, people who are not trained in first aid or medical professions may be exempted from the legal obligation to offer emergency help.

But this does not mean that one can simply leave a casualty whom they know is in danger. Doing so may make you liable through your omission to act.

If you are not capable of providing skilled emergency assistance, take the following steps in the event someone suffers a life-threatening injury:

- Call for an ambulance, fire service or police
- Protect the injured from further harm
- Position the injured properly so that they can breathe
- Provide comfort

The advices above are not intended to frighten or deter a potential Good Samaritan, but rather to inform potential rescuers of the current legal situation.

COUNTER TERRORISM

Kenya has been a fertile ground for series of severe terror attacks, often carried out in populous cities such as Nairobi as well as coastal and northern counties.

August 7, 2008 bombing of the US embassy in Nairobi remains the deadliest in Kenya's history. 213 people were killed, while at least 4,000 more were injured.

In April 2015, students at Garissa University College were attacked by Al-Shabaab gunmen. At least 148 were massacred, in what was described as the second worst terror attack in Kenyan history.

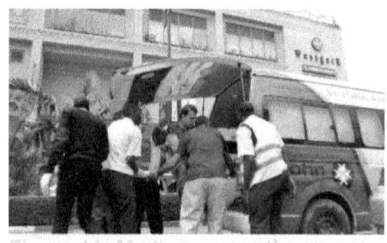

Figure 11: Medics evacuating a casualty with gunshot wound from the Westgate Mall

In another horrific attack, the group killed 67 people during a four-day siege at Westgate shopping mall in the capital, Nairobi, in September 2013.

Following the spate of attacks, many people now live in fear spread over further promised retaliations.

Terrorism is described as the unofficial or unauthorized use of violence and intimidation to cause fear in the pursuit of political aims.

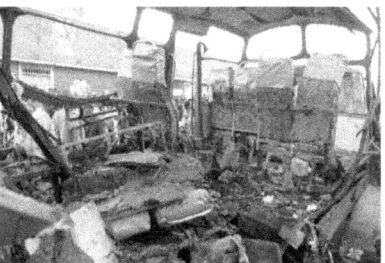

Even though everyone is vulnerable, crowded places such as schools, churches, pubs, and matatus (public vehicles) are sensitive hotspots due to unsuspecting huge masses.

Figure 12: At least five people were killed and 18 others seriously injured in a grenade attack in Nairobi's Eastleigh estate

During such incidents of terror attacks, people find it easy to point an accusing finger to the ill-preparedness of the security agencies to deal with the nagging attackers.

But one thing that the whole world agrees is that security begins with everyone.

As security agencies are working hard to put their acts together, each person can play a role in securing the public spaces.

2.1 | Mitigating Terrorism Threats

C ivilians are the first line of defense in protecting fellow citizens from the threat of terror attacks. Be aware and report suspicious activity by calling hotlines immediately.

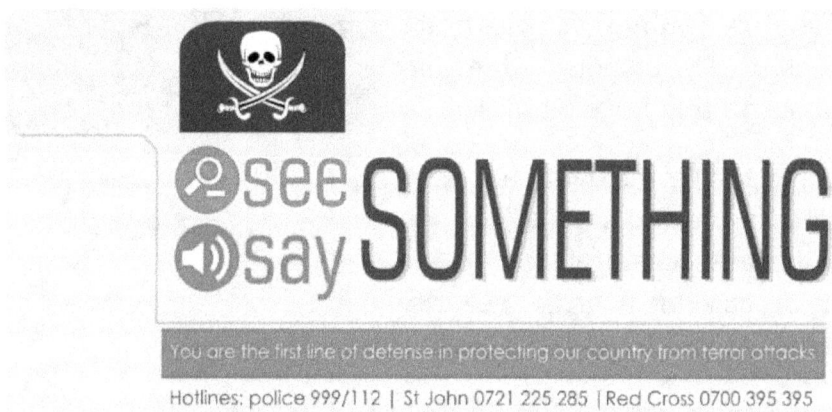

see **SOMETHING**
say

You are the first line of defense in protecting our country from terror attacks

Hotlines: police 999/112 | St John 0721 225 285 | Red Cross 0700 395 395

The following key points summarize some behaviors that could be suspicious:

- ➲ Abnormal packages: Unattended packages, generally small and easily transportable improvised explosive devices.
- ➲ Surveillance: Photographing entrances, exits, or security measures, as well as asking inappropriate questions about the facility and its security. This is done during the planning phase by terrorists.

- **Abnormal or Bulky Clothing:** Clothing that is too warm for the season. Unusually thick clothing could be used to conceal weapons.
- **Unauthorized Entrance into Restricted Areas:** Persons sneaking into restricted areas or following others into locked buildings.
- **Suspicious Vehicles:** Vehicles apparently left vacant for long periods, or vehicles parked in prohibited areas.

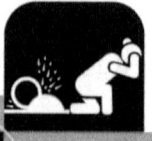

2.2 | Surviving Terror Attacks

Explosives

A hand grenade is one of the most common explosive weapons used by terrorists. It takes about 5 seconds to go off. So you still have a little time to act.

In case an explosive is hulled near you, it should be your natural instinct to lie down on your stomach and protect eardrums using your fingers.

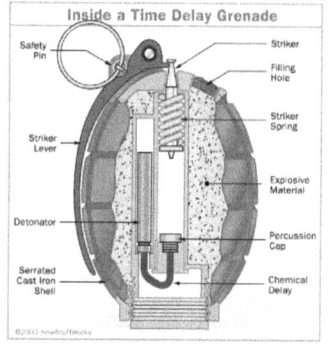

Cross your feet with legs pointing towards the explosive because they are not as fatal like other parts of the body.

Lying down minimizes the body surface exposed, as fragments mostly fly at an angle of above 40 degrees.

However, do not lie on the ground for too long. Lie down for about 10 seconds, then take off before you become vulnerable to secondary attacks by terrorists.

Do not run when an explosive is hurled towards you. You won't run faster than the fragments. And the impact of the explosion will blow you off your feet and throw you to a wall maybe. You also expose yourself to be hit by the fragments.

In a building explosion, vacate quickly and calmly. If unable to leave, get under a strong desk to avoid falling items.

Gun Attacks

In some instances, an active shooting event immediately follows after the explosion.

An active shooter is a terrorist actively engaged in killing or attempting to kill people in a confined and populated area, typically through the use of firearms.

Victims are selected at random or profiled on certain criteria. The event is unpredictable, evolves quickly, and law enforcement is usually required to end an active shooter event.

When an active shooter is in your vicinity, you must be prepared both mentally and physically to deal with the situation. You have three options: Run, hide, or fight as a last resort.

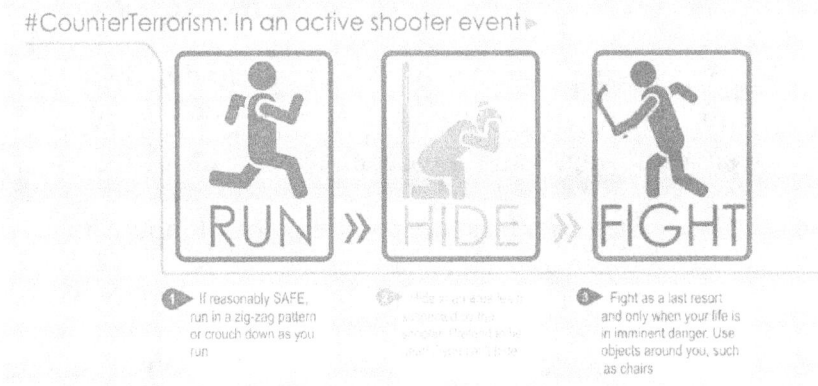

#CounterTerrorism: In an active shooter event

RUN » HIDE » FIGHT

1. If reasonably SAFE, run in a zig-zag pattern or crouch down as you run

2. Hide in a quiet area

3. Fight as a last resort and only when your life is in imminent danger. Use objects around you, such as chairs

Run

- If reasonably safe, run in a zig-zag pattern or crouch down as you run. If not, you need to hide and barricade yourself.

- Have an escape route and plan in mind.

- Leave your belongings behind.

- Help others escape, if possible.

- Evacuate regardless of whether others agree to follow.

- Prevent others from entering an area where the active shooter may be.

- Call the police hotlines (999 or 112)* when you are safe.

NOTE: *Sometimes these hotlines may not be working or busy, therefore, you may need to have alternative office lines.

Hide

- As tempting as it may be during shootouts, do not take off when it's not safe. Seek cover, survey the surroundings and then decide your next move.

- Hide in an area least suspected by the shooter.

- Lock the door or block the entry to your hiding place.

- Silence your cell phone (including the vibrate mode) and remain quiet.

- Consider pretending to be dead if you can't hide yourself.

Fight

- When facing an armed attacker, you need to control your adrenaline rush, understand the weapon, and initiate a clear plan of action.

- Your plan of action should usually be to run or hide. Fight only as a last resort if you are cornered and have no means of escape.

- While fighting, attempt to incapacitate the shooter using improvised weapons around you, such as chairs, fire extinguisher, or bottle. Act with as much physical aggression as possible and commit to your actions. Your life depends on it.

- You can also attempt to disarm the assailant. But remember it has a high risk of injury or death.

- When disarming, the first thing to control is the weapon by snatching the gun out of the attacker's hands.

- If the attacker is pointing the gun at your face, (1) you may pretend to be raising your arms, (2) move away from the shooting path, and (3) grasp the barrel of the gun from underneath and twist upwards. The three moves should be done in a split second.

- Once you reach for the gun, incapacitate the attacker by hitting soft-spots, such as groin, sternum, adam's apple, or pock eyes with your fingers.

2.4 | Cooperating with Security Agencies

L aw enforcement is usually required to end an active shooting event.

The first officers to arrive to the scene may not stop to help injured persons. Expect rescue teams to follow the initial officers. These rescue teams will treat and remove the injured.

During the operation, observe the following:

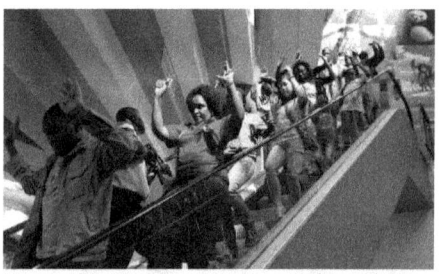

Figure 13: Hostages walk to safety with their hands up during Westgate Mall terror attack

- Do not leave the area until law enforcement authorities instruct you to do so.

- Always stop and remain still when contacted by police at crime scene. Any unexpected movement you make is one step closer to getting shot, especially hand movements.

- Do what you're told by Police, and do it slowly. e.g. lie down, carry up your hands.

- Never flee from armed police. Doing this arouses suspicion and greatly increases the chance of a fatal misunderstanding.

- Let yourself be handcuffed at crime scene. It is police protocol to place handcuffs on even the most cooperative of suspects.

- Put down any item in your hand such as bags or jackets, and show the police officer your open hands at crime scene. This will reduce their fear that you have a concealed weapon.

- Keep hands visible at all times.

- Avoid quick movements toward officers such as holding on to them for safety.

- Do not attempt to fight off a police officer. Assaulting him will most certainly get you a place in jail or send you to your maker.

- If you are carrying a firearm at crime scene, take care not to point it at a police officer. Doing so could make the officer shoot you.

- Avoid threatening police officers or describing what your friends or family might do in retaliation for their actions. This will only make things worse for you.

Once you have reached a safe location, you will likely be held in that area by law enforcement until the situation is under control, and all witnesses have been identified and questioned.

CRIME PREVENTION AND SAFETY

Increasing incidences of crime across the country are becoming a matter of grave concern.

Of even greater concern is that a number of these crimes go unreported, encouraging the so called 'petty criminals' to advance to sophisticated crime as they have no fear of being apprehended.

In the daily lives of Kenyans, handbags and jewelry are snatched. Stealing of mobile phones and computers is also so common that citizens just do not consider reporting the crime.

The same position prevails in the cases of sexual offences, where the victims and their families do not report cases due to the very nature of the offences which can and does stigmatize the victim.

However, the most common crimes are break-ins and carjacking, with the stolen cars used by the criminals to commit armed robberies. "Snatch and run" crimes are also becoming more common on city streets.

A young lady cannot have a walk in town at midnight without fear of being molested and motorists drive with fear of their side mirrors and lights being ripped off their cars.

But the biggest and most profound culprits of hiding criminal activities of massive scale takes place by bankers and other corporate bodies who, for the sake of their corporate image, condone white-collar crimes.

And then come the in-house banking scams. It is an acknowledged reality within the banking industry that colossal frauds, mostly related with cyber-crimes, take place and the banks do not report or even pursue the criminals.

Recently, a local bank lost close to Sh200 million and when the culprits were discovered, the bank struck a deal with the offenders to refund part of the loot. No report to the police, no investigations, no punishment of the offenders!

A Kenya Cyber security report by Serianu Company notes that Kenyan companies lost over Sh15 billion in 2015 through Cybercrime.

More worrying is that 22 million mobile phone subscribers access and are constantly on the internet, but doesn't have mobile security in place.

This is a huge vulnerability gap, considering that mobile transactions have become the most convenient way of banking through USSDs, short codes and mobile apps.

An Economic Survey shows that criminal activities in Kenya continued to grow, with 72,490 cases reported in 2015, compared to 69,376 in 2014 and 71,832 in 2013.

The report shows that Kiambu County had the highest number of reported crime cases at 4,768, followed by Nakuru (4,384), Nairobi (4,383), Meru (4,215), and Mombasa (3,194). In 2015, the most prevalent crime counties were Nairobi (6,732 incidents), Nakuru (4,525), and Kiambu (4,449).

Even though these annual crime statistics are best practices across the world, they are not a true reflection, bearing in mind the wave of crimes which go unreported and therefore unaddressed by the investigative and prosecutorial agencies.

On the other side, police do not have the capacity to investigate every crime. In Nairobi's poor neighborhoods, gangs have taken over the provision of security, charging residents a fee. Slum residents prefer these gangs because they solve cases faster than the police.

3.1 Crime Hotspots

Security researchers have mapped out crime hotspots where you are likely to be attacked by criminals and possibly get killed. Some of the hotspots are:

- City Cotton between Wilson Airport and South C - Common for murder and mugging.
- Mathare Slum area near Oilibya Petrol Station - Common for mugging and murder crimes.
- Congo area near Kawangware - Common for drug trafficking, rape and mugging.
- Kware in Rongai, Kajiado - Common for mugging crimes.
- Noonkopir (Daraja next to Saitoti Hospital) in Kitengela -Common for carjacking and robbery.
- Kiwanja ya Punda (around Migoni House) in Kiserian - Common for rape and murder crimes.
- Around Kiserian Primary - Common for carjacking and murder.
- Kisaju road stretch in Isinya - Common for carjacking and rape crimes.
- Kichinjio area in Isinya - Common for murder and rape.
- Kiandutu area in Thika - Common for assaults, break-ins, arson and drug trafficking crimes.
- Mangu flyover in Thika - Common for robbery and mugging.

- Railway (Nairobi-Nakuru Highway junction to Kikuyu town) - Common for rape, murder and carjacking.
- Across Patel bridge in Kikuyu - Common for murder.
- Kiandutu slums in Kikuyu- Common for robbery and rape.
- Mashimoni (Marimari) road in Kiambu - Common for carjacking, robbery and mugging.
- Limuru road stretch between the town and the Nakuru Highway - Common for carjacking and mugging.
- Kisumu Ndogo area in Athi River - Common for murder crimes and mugging.
- Kosovo in Athi River - Common for robbery and mugging.
- Behind Muli block in Mlolongo - Common for rape and mugging crimes.
- Madharau Street in Mlolongo - Common for rape and robbery.
- Near Silanga dam in Mlolongo - Common for murder and assault.
- Kona Mbaya in Ruai - Common for mugging and rape.
- Sewage area along Maji Mazuri road, Ruai - Common for murder and rape.

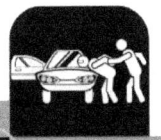

3.2 | Survive Carjacking

Carjacking, by a group of people who always think they have the right to what someone else owns, is one of the most common crimes in Kenya.

These criminals seek easy access to vehicles, making carjacking a crime of opportunity, preventable by simple deterrents, such as keeping doors and windows closed whether you are in the car or not.

If you think a carjacker is trailing you, make a few turns to confirm if they are indeed following you, drive to the police or area with people.

Give up your car keys and leave the scene if you're confronted by armed carjacker. You can get another car, but not another life.

Without being obvious, try to get a description of the carjacker's age, sex, height, hair color, clothes, etc.

Immediately after you get away from the carjacker or he drives off, call the police.

To ensure security of the vehicle:

⮑ Try to park in well lit, open areas, and in view of a security camera.

- Never leave valuable items out in the open in a vehicle. Either remove them from the car or place inside the glove box, under seats, or in the trunk where others cannot see them.

- While driving, keep doors and windows locked to prevent a carjacking. Also, always lock car doors when leaving a vehicle.

- When walking back to a parked car, look underneath vehicle and in back seat after entering a car to make sure no one is under or in the car.

- Do not leave helmet or riding equipment with a motorcycle after parking it.

- Chain and lock motorcycle to a secure unmovable item when leaving it unattended.

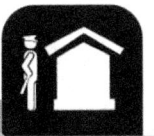

3.3 Domestic Security

While it's difficult to protect your home from professional thieves, most home burglaries are done by amateurs. The following quick guide can help you thwart these thieves:

- lock all doors and windows, even if leaving the house for a short time.

- Never let anyone know that there is nobody in a house by posting leading information on social media.

- Provide visibility around the house by ensuring that there are no dark, hiding areas around the house.

- Trim trees surrounding the house so that burglars do not have easy access to the roof.

- Consider getting a dog as a pet to scare away strangers or a CCTV camera that can be accessed remotely.

- Be wary of solicitors trying to get information on your day to day routine in order to burglarize your home.

- If you're going away, use timers for television and radio to make the house appear as if it is currently occupied. Unplug all non-essential electronics that could get blown, and close all the water taps, you may return to a flooded house.

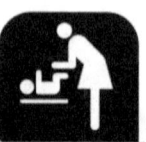

3.4 | Safeguarding Children

It might be difficult to accept, but every child can be kidnapped, hurt, or abused sexually. The following basic precautions can help keep your kids away from dangers:

- ⊃ Teach your kid to avoid talking to strangers, unless they need help from "safe" stranger like police.

- ⊃ Never let your kid go anywhere alone. Another trusted adult should be present if you cannot.

- ⊃ Know what your children wear every day. Avoid putting their names on the outside of their clothes. Children may respond more readily to a stranger who calls them by name.

- ⊃ Never leave your child alone in a vehicle, restroom, store, playground, or other public place.

- ⊃ Keep updated information of your children's pictures, identifying marks, medical records, etc.

- ⊃ Find out why your child doesn't want to be with someone or go somewhere. The reason may be more than a personality conflict or a lack of interest.

- ⊃ Encourage your child to tell you about what makes them uncomfortable, or scares them. Listen to what they say and never underestimate their concerns.

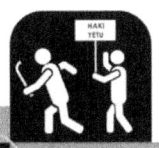

3.5 | Surviving Violent Mobs

A ngry and violent mobs can be just as dangerous and unpredictable as any other natural disaster. Post-election violence of December 2007 exemplified how worse these violence can be. About 1,500 people were killed and 600,000 displaced after the disputed presidential election.

There has also been minor skirmishes, which have cumulatively resulted into many fatalities and displacements. The major reasons fueling these ethnic conflicts are unresolved border disputes, cattle rustling, competition over land and water resources, and political conflict.

Violent mobs are also witnessed in the aftermath of football events. The most notorious are Gor Mahia and AFC Leopards football fans, who have recently intensified violence and destruction of property, 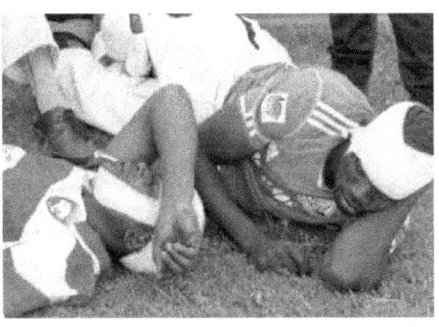 every time their teams take to the field to clash in mouthwatering encounters.

Protesting students also engage in street confrontation with anti-riot police, blocking busy highways and major roads.

The following guidelines could help you avoid or escape such violent mobs:

- If there is no obvious danger like stoning, stay calm and walk at all times. If you run or move too quickly, you might attract unwanted attention.

- Unless your car is the focus for the angry mob, continue driving as calmly as possible.

- Do not wear clothing that could be interpreted as provocative, military or police wear.

- Do not try to confront rioters or looters to prevent property damage. No material thing is worth your life.

- If you're on foot, move away by going with the flow of foot traffic, not against it to avoid being trampled on.

- Have ID and emergency contact information on you in case you are arrested or become unconscious.

- Secure your home or business and get risk insurance if rioting is imminent.

- Make sure you know several routes for getting and leaving home.

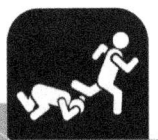

3.6 | Safety Actions during Stampedes

In a crowded or mob situation, it is easy to stumble and fall to the ground, increasing the chances of being trampled as crowds begin to stampede.

Whenever you are in a crowded venue, such as stadium, rallies, concert halls, always take a mental note of the location of the exits.

If you find yourself in the middle of a moving crowd, move away by going with the flow of foot traffic, not against it to avoid being trampled on.

Zigzag towards exit with your hands up to protect your chest and head, taking advantage of any space that may open up to move sideways.

If you fall, get up quickly or keep moving by crawling in the same direction of the crowd, or cover your head with arms and lie on your side drawing in your legs.

The worst scenario is to be pushed by the crowd against an immovable object. Try to stay away from walls or barricades.

3.7 Mitigating Workplace Violence

Workplace violence and harassment are serious and potentially costly issues, that can affect the safety of every employee and business, regardless of sector or occupation.

In recognition of this fact the following steps would help reduce the risk:

- Screening workers before hiring, to obtain a thorough work history, criminal record and references from sources you develop - not just those supplied.

- Initiate employee assistance programs to provide treatment for emotional, marital, substance abuse and financial problems.

- Train workers in conflict resolution and stress management techniques.

- Increase the perception of surveillance in all rooms and entrances.

- Put in place a zero tolerance policy for drugs, violence and harassment in the workplace.

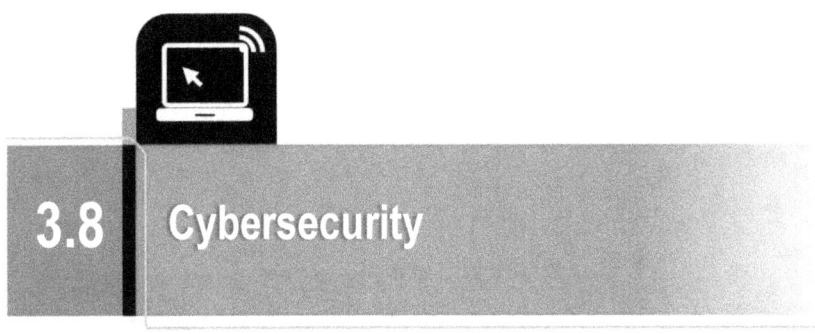

3.8 Cybersecurity

Cybersecurity in Kenya is the single biggest concern to banks in terms of the consumption and use of Information Communication Technologies (ICT).

Whereas banks may have invested heavily in ICT security systems, most Kenyans remain grossly unaware of the various cyber security threats that exist.

Some key principles of safer online banking and payments to consider include using trust-worthy devices and internet connections, while keeping the operating systems and software up-to-date.

Not every internet connection such as public Wi-Fi is secure to be used for online banking or making payments. It is advisable instead to use a virtual private network (VPN) to keep your communications encrypted (unreadable) to anyone who may try to intercept them.

Whenever you connect to your online account, use your own computer, tablet or smartphone as it is more likely to notice if any suspicious activity is going. Avoid using a borrowed or public device that might put your data, account or savings at risk.

But having a strong password is perhaps the first step in proactively securing your device and online banking access.

It is even more important never to reuse your password e.g. for your bank, social media and other accounts which can mean a total hack into each account in case it leaks from any one of them.

there is also influx of "Dating Websites," with potential victims of romance scam already identified for the scammers, including hints on the type of person they want to fall in love with, the location and age range. To prevent:

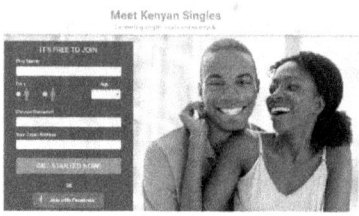
Figure 14: Typical Dating Site

- ⤳ Don't send money through the bank or mobile money transfer to a person you have never personally met.

- ⤳ Beware of someone you never met who wants a statement of money erroneously sent to you and wants refund to his mobile or bank account.

- ⤳ Like any scam use your computer to your advantage. There are mobile apps and websites, such as truecaller.com, that can help you identify the person for arrest by police.

FIRE SAFETY

Fire is one of the most frequent disaster in Kenya. A week barely passes before a fire incident is reported, mostly in congested slums.

These informal settlements have become a death trap for many people, some of whom have died in mysterious fire disasters.

The most horrible was the Sinai fire tragedy in September 2011, where as many as 120 people were burned beyond recognition when a pipeline burst into flames as slum dwellers were siphoning fuel from it.

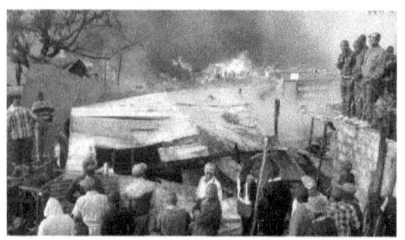

Figure 15: Firefighters battling inferno as millions of property go into flames at Gikomba Market in Nairobi

In slums, fire engines are in many occasions reduced to mere spectators, extinguishing flames at the periphery, as there is no access roads and every square inch of land is occupied.

Causes of such urban fires include electrical faults and burst paraffin stoves or overturned tin lamps and candles.

This worrying trend of fatal fire disasters is also creeping into schools.

Among the cases that stirred the nation's conscience over the years was one involving Moi Girls High School in Nairobi in 2017, where 10 girls died in dormitory fire. In 2001, 68 boys were burnt to death at Kyanguli Secondary School in Machakos. In the same year at Bombolulu Girls in Mombasa, 58 children died in a dormitory fire. Earlier in 1991 and 1999, 19 girls and four boys died in separate school fire incidents at St Kizito and Nyeri High Schools respectively.

In 2016, at least 126 schools were burnt in a wave of fires. The major causes of such fires include electrical faults and arson attacks by disgruntled students.

In an attempt to curb these incidents, education ministry developed a safety manual, outlining guidelines on issues like disaster preparedness, school-community relations, safe structure, and how to create a conducive teaching and learning environment among others.

However, despite these advances, the country is still grappling with the challenge of occasional incidents of school fires.

Fire cannot start, unless all these four elements are present – fuel, oxygen, heat, and chemical reaction.

Therefore, the basic principle for extinguishment of fire is eliminating any of the four elements, except fuel which is not practical to remove.

Due to its nature of spreading fast before fire engines arrive, people need to learn basic ways of putting out fires.

Local materials, such as water, sand, or soaked blanket, can be used to put out fire from ordinary combustibles if fire extinguishers are not available.

However, the perfect way to put out fire is to use extinguishers, classified on the basis of the type of fire as described below:

- *Ordinary combustibles, such as wood, paper, and fabric* - extinguished by any fire extinguisher, except CO_2.

- *Flammable liquids, such as petroleum* - extinguished by foam, dry powder, or CO_2 extinguisher, but not water.

- *Combustible gases, such as cooking gas* - extinguished by dry powder.

- *Electrical fires, mainly caused by short-circuiting or overloading of electrical cables* - extinguished by CO2 or dry powder extinguisher only.

- *Combustible metals, such as potassium or sodium* - extinguished by dry powder only.

- *Unsaturated cooking oils and fats in the kitchen* - extinguishable by fire blanket or wet chemical extinguisher only.

There is no universal fire extinguishing agent, though dry powder can be used to put out almost all fires. The guide below assist in selecting the most effective fire extinguishing agent:

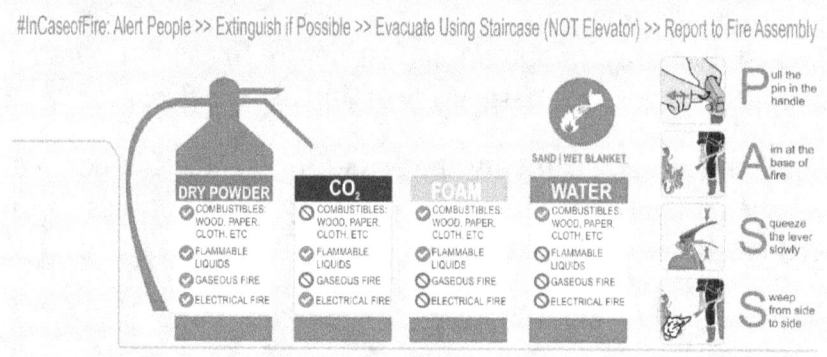

#InCaseofFire: Alert People >> Extinguish if Possible >> Evacuate Using Staircase (NOT Elevator) >> Report to Fire Assembly

Fire ball extinguisher is also one of the new fastest and efficient way of extinguishing fire. When thrown into fire it explodes.

4.2 | Action during Fire Outbreaks

It is important to take precautions to prevent fire outbreaks. However, fire may still occur even when you try to prevent it. Therefore, you may need to take an insurance cover against fire risks.

Meanwhile, the following guidelines can help you know what to do if one should break out.

Evacuation procedure

- Alert people by shouting or pressing the bell.

- Extinguish if possible, without risking your life.

- Evacuate everyone using the staircase, not elevators.

- Close door (do not lock) in each room after escaping.

- Feel doors before opening, and do not open a door that is hot.

- Do not throw water on an electrical or petroleum fire.

- Refer serious first aid emergencies to trained First Aiders or ambulance responders.

- Assemble at the designated fire assembly point.

Action when cloth is on fire

#FireSafety: Action when cloth is on fire ▶

STOP ≫ DROP ≫ ROLL

STOP, DROP, and ROLL if clothing catches fire to avoid fanning the flames

Action when caught in smoke filled room

- If the room is smoky, lie low near the floor where there is more oxygen, and scroll towards window.

- If you cannot escape a building on fire, seal door openings and cracks with wet clothing, and call firefighters, giving your exact location

- Jump through the window as a last resort, with legs first.

- If you cannot escape a building on fire, staff clothing to seal door cracks and call firefighters, giving your exact location.

4.3 Preventing Fire Hazards

H azards are threats to fire safety, such as a situation that increases the likelihood of a fire or may impede escape in the event a fire occurs.

Take the following precautions to prevent ignition of fire, limit its development, or effects after it starts:

- Install smoke detectors and replace batteries at least once in six months.

- Never allow smoke in a bed or sleeping room.

- Keep curtains and other flammable objects away from fireplaces and stoves.

- Keep a fire extinguisher in the kitchen and know how to use it.

- Tie back long hair or loose clothing when cooking.

- Do not hold an infant when cooking or drinking a hot liquid.

- Avoid cooking when sleeping or taking medications.

- Read direction before using household chemicals, and keep all products in their original containers.

- Ensure adequate ventilation when using chemicals with dangerous fumes and protect hands with heavy gloves.

- Store ignition sources such as matches, lighters, and candles away from children.

- Plan escape route, teach children where to go if fire breaks out.

- Never store flammable substances, such as petrol, in house.

- Conduct fire drills to test level of preparedness.

4.4 | Preventing Electrocution

E lectrical shock effects can range from a slight tingling to instant death. The severity of an electrocution injury depends on the voltage.

To prevent chances of electrocution:

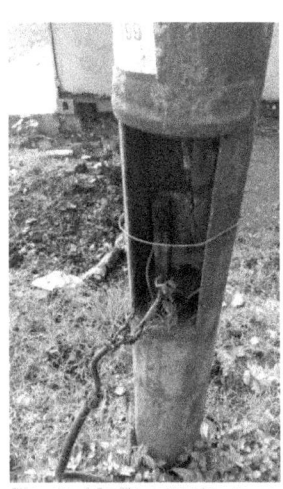

Figure 16: Exposed electric wires on street light pole can cause electrocution during rainy seasons.

- ⤷ Repair damaged appliances, wiring, cords, and plugs.

- ⤷ Never use electrical appliances anywhere they might come in contact with water.

- ⤷ Keep children away from electric appliances and teach them about the dangers of electricity as soon as they are old enough.

- ⤷ Check power cords attached to electrical appliances and extension cords making sure there are no loose or exposed wires.

- ⤷ Don't use electrical appliances in wet locations or allow them to get wet.

- ⤷ Don't overload power outlets by plugging in too many appliances.

- Switch off appliances like microwave if food catches fire.

- Never forget - water and electricity don't mix.

- Avoid touching a person being electrocuted, you will get an electric shock too, and may also be injured.

In case a victim suffers electrical shock, disable the power, check if casualty is conscious. People who have been electrocuted are likely to have breathing problems and heart failure. Administer heart resuscitation if casualty is not breathing.

Chapter 5

HEAVY RAIN AND FLOOD RESILIENCE

Heavy downpour that pounds various parts of the country during short rains (October-December) and long rains (March-May) has the likelihood of causing serious incidents of flooding and other trail of damages.

In urban areas, there are incidents of terrible traffic jams, and commuters spending nights in their cars due to impassable roads.

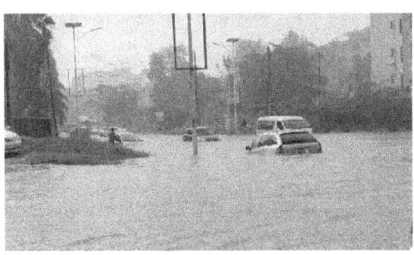

Figure 17: Section of Ojijo Road in Parklands rendered impassable as heavy floods ran on the roads following heavy downpour in Nairobi

Lives are lost by drowning, electrocution, landslide, flooding in homes, and poorly built structures collapse.

The Meteorological Department always sound the alarm of looming period of heavy rainfall.

Following these announcements, Kenyans react in varied ways. Some ignore the alerts, arguing that they are routine lies and inaccurate forecasts by the weatherman. Others are worried of the potential dangers that come with heavy downpours, including terrible traffic jams, drowning and lightning strike among others.

Of course whether the rains pour as predicted or not is debatable, however, everyone need to be prepared for likely calamities.

During these incidents, some people find it easy to point an accusing finger to the ill-preparedness of the authorities in dealing with rain and flood related calamities.

But one thing that the whole world agrees is that safety begins with everyone. As authorities are trying to put their acts together, each person can play a role in improving their personal preparedness to deal with common emergencies around them.

Floods and flash floods

For instance, those living in flood-prone areas can take necessary steps like moving to safer grounds, reinforcing weak walls and unblocking household drainage systems.

However, the only noticeable preparedness step taken by many Kenyans in such circumstance is the buying of umbrellas from the streets and local supermarkets.

The fact that government has the primary responsibility to protect its citizens is not disputable. But residents, who bear the biggest burden of loss, can also make a difference.

It is worrying that most of the drowning cases reported in the past occurred as a result of people underestimating the strength of moving water, ignoring simple safety advices with fatal consequences.

For instance, pedestrians and motorists are swept while attempting to cross swollen rivers that overflow over bridges despite knowing that others have died in similar circumstances.

They are senselessly walking or driving to their deaths, instead of being patient for water levels to subside.

Walking in floodwaters is dangerous, not only because of the likelihood of being swept downstream; you can also get contamination by raw sewage or electrocuted by electrically charged waterway. Venomous snakes may also bite you!

In rare occasions, you may be caught up in the middle of floods, and have to move in water. A less risky action in such a situation is to:

- Walk where the water is not rising above your knee level. You can use a stick to check the ground in front of you, as water can be much deeper than it appears.
- For those evacuating in a car, drive through as little water as possible, and take the shortest route to a safe parking.
- Without hesitation, abandon your car immediately if it stalls in rapidly rising waters, and climb to higher ground. Your life is more important and irreplaceable, unlike your car.
- While escaping, the door may not open due to pressure from the water outside the car. For this reason, quickly use the windows to escape before the car's electronic system fails.

When it comes to giving first aid for a near-drowning casualty;

- Check for breathing and other signs of life.
- If the victim is unconscious but breathing, lay him in a slightly tilted position, with the head and mouth on the lower side to allow water drain off by gravity. Be ready to resuscitate in case they are not breathing.
- Do not press the victim's stomach to drain swallowed water. This may force water to block the lung vessels, preventing intake of oxygen.
- In cold weather drowning, remove the victim's wet clothing and cover with a blanket or worm clothing. To boost warming, you can give them chocolate or hot drinks, but not energy drink.

Collapsing buildings

Collapsing structures is another calamity which people need to watch out for during the rainy season. The incidents are likely to occur in urban areas like Nairobi, Mombasa, Kisii and Kisumu, where similar incidences have occurred in the past.

Most of these structures cave in due to poor workmanship or use of substandard materials that cannot withstand seepage from heavy rains.

The developers also change the approved designs to accommodate their own selfish interests, endangering the lives of tenants.

So, before getting buried in the debris, here are the tell-tale signs of imminent structural collapse to worry about and vacate:

- Building constructed too close to a waterway
- Structural cracks, mostly leading to foundation

- Flats that go beyond four flours without an elevator

- Water seeping from walls and ever-flooded basement

- Weird crack sounds, especially during strong winds

- Flats partly occupied and upper floors under construction

You can consult an expert in case you notice your building has most of these tell-tale signs, as its better to be safe than sorry!

But more sustainably, the Government needs to enforce policies and laws controlling urban development, especially those close to waterways.

However, the enforcement has been met with minimal success. But as the Government gets its act together, everyone needs to play their part.

Regardless of what causes the collapse, there are ways to survive and escape death or severe injury.

Usually, the collapse occurs very quickly, leaving you with a few seconds for quick action.

When you notice that the wall is caving in and you cannot get out in time; position yourself next to a sturdy piece of furniture such as heavy desk, sofa, or large overstuffed armchair, lying on the floor in foetal position.

The furniture may be able to support the weight of a collapsing wall and create a triangular space adjacent to it where you will be relatively safe. In this position, you may get injured, but chances are that you're likely to come out of the wreckage alive.

Once the building has finished collapsing and there is no more movement, then it is time to carefully assess the situation.

If you have an electronic device of any kind with a cellular signal, use it. If not, stay where you are and call loudly for help.

However, do not waste all of your energy screaming after you see that nobody is coming anytime soon. Instead, conserve your energy and use it only when you hear a rescue team is near.

If you find that you are having trouble breathing, cup your hands over your nose and mouth and breathe into them.

In case you are wounded, stop the bleeding by applying pressure using your hand, bandage or clean cloth.

Electrocution

Electrocution is also common during heavy downpours. It is typically caused by pools of water, fence, or clothesline accidentally connected to live electricity wires.

To prevent such chances of being electrocuted, never forget that water and electricity don't mix.

Hence, avoid needless touching of streetlight pole, wired fence or clothesline which is likely to be connected to electricity in a nearby building.

Also avoid stepping on pools of water without insulated shoes like gumboots.

If you notice a person being electrocuted, never touch them as you will get an electric shock too. Instead, use a non-conductor material like dry wood or plastic to remove the connection to electricity and switch off power where possible.

People who have been electrocuted are likely to have breathing problems and heart failure. After power is switched off, give two rescue breaths followed by 30 chest compressions if there is no breathing

Other soft tissue injuries can be treated by detecting entrance wound, usually dry and leathery, and exit wound, which is much larger, and cover the burn with dry, loose, non-sticky dressing.

The severity of an electrocution injury depends on the voltage. Shock from high voltage power lines can jump up to 18 meters and will nearly always kill instantly.

In such high voltage electrocution, call Kenya Power on 95551 or 0703070707 to switch off power before starting to offer first aid.

Lightning

Another likely cause of electrocution during stormy rains is lightning strikes, which is very common in western Kenya, especially in Kisii, Kisumu, Kakamega and Bungoma counties.

To escape such strikes, try to find shelter in a building during a lightning storm, and if indoors, keep away from windows.

If no shelter is available, try to be the lowest object around, but avoid sheltering under lone tree or stepping on water.

First aid for lightning and electrical burns are similar, and all the injuries should be evaluated in hospital for possible damage to internal organs like lung or heart.

Road carnage

Another danger that people have to contend with during periods of heavy downpours are road accidents resulting from poor visibility and slippery roads.

In these situations, motorists need to drive at a speed that allows them to spot hazards and react accordingly.

They should avoid dangerous overtaking and distracted driving activities such as using a cell phone or stealing a quick glance at an attractive pedestrian.

In addition, motorist need to desist from the temptation of driving on free gear to save fuel. It's difficult to re-engage brakes or gears when free-wheeling downhill, leading to fatal accidents.

Charcoal jiko poisoning

Finally, there can be avoidable instances of carbon monoxide poisoning, mostly from using charcoal jikos for warming an enclosed room on a cold night. The gas is lethal and termed as 'silent killer' because it's invisible, odourless, and tasteless.

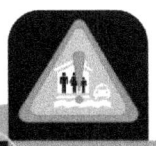

5.1 Flood Hotspots

Some of the areas which have been worst hit by floods in the recent past include:

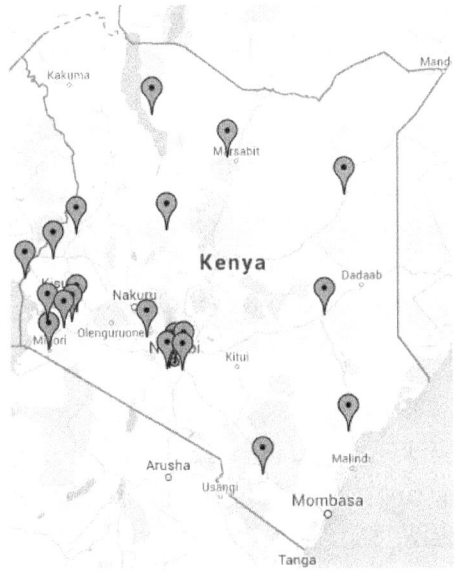

- Wajir
- Trans Nzoia
- Maralal
- Garissa
- Nairobi, Mathare
- Ong'ata Rongai
- Kiserian
- Ruai
- Athi River
- Samburu
- Migori
- Homabay
- Nyakach
- Kisii
- Bungoma
- Busia
- Taita Taveta
- Tana River

- Narok
- Mount Elgon
- Isiolo
- Voi

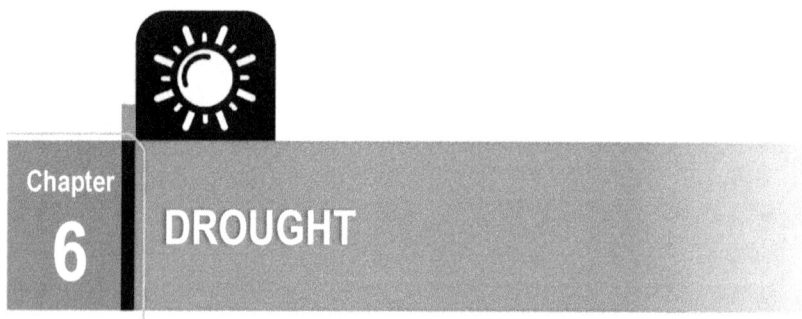

Chapter 6 | DROUGHT

Millions of Kenyans are each time left on the brink of starvation whenever there is prolonged drought and erratic rains, affecting food production.

Most of those at risk are small-scale herders in arid and semi-arid lands, where livestock rearing account for as much as 90 percent of family income.

Northern Kenya, parts of eastern, coastal region and Rift Valley are the most affected areas.

These dry areas are home to approximately 30 percent (12 million) of Kenya's people and 50 percent of its livestock.

In urban areas, however, where thousands have flocked in search of hard-to-come by jobs, hunger ravages families not because there is no food to buy, but people cannot afford.

Prices of most basic foods that include maize flour, sukuma wiki, and rice escalate due to prevailing drought conditions, making them inaccessible.

For instance in Nairobi, 60 percent of people stay in slums, doing erratic jobs and cannot afford three proper meals a day, amid rising food prices. Some do away with lunch in their houses because they cannot afford it.

Many school children in these dingy slums take only porridge for breakfast, lunch and supper. If things are better they get a mixture of beans and maize from a roadside kiosk.

6.1 Causes and Impact of Drought

Forest damage and emission of carbon fumes are the root causes of increasing global temperatures and ensuing drought in Kenya.

However, the situation is aggravated by overdependence on rainfall, yet the country is water scarce, with per capita water availability being one of the lowest in Africa.

Agriculture, which is the backbone of the county's economy, is almost entirely rain-fed.

Water for human consumption and other uses is derived from rivers whose recharge depends on rainfall.

As a result, drought undesirably affects all sectors of the economy and the population at large. Some of the impacts include;

- Crop failures, leading to reduced food security.

- Deaths of humans, livestock and wildlife due to lack of food and pasture.

- Cost of basic food stuffs like maize and beans rise beyond reach of many households.

- Deterioration of human and animal health as a result of malnutrition and poor access to quality water.

- Conflicts arise between communities and wildlife over grazing lands.

- The ravaging hunger triggers school closures.

- People living in urban areas experience rationing of water and electricity power.

- Workers lose jobs when industries shut down as raw materials get depleted.

- Scorching effect of droughts also leads to environmental degradation and desertification.

6.2 Drought Adaptation and Coping Mechanisms

With the rising cases of drought as the world heats, the time has come where mitigating future climate change must be accompanied by adapting to the climate change already caused. Doing nothing will be dangerous.

As a long-term solution, planting trees is vital in adapting to global warming and combating drought by influencing rainfall patterns.

The trees take water from the soil and release it into the atmosphere. Tree leaves also remove carbon dioxide from the atmosphere.

But, the following adaptation and coping mechanisms are also key in averting the losses and impacts of draught during the onset:

- ⮑ Take famine early warning systems seriously, as it assesses food security, mainly in vulnerable areas.

- ⮑ Use irrigation and rainfall alternately for crop farming.

- ⮑ If you can afford, do greenhouse farming.

- ⮑ Plant drought tolerant crops like melons, millet, cassava, and cowpea.

- ⮑ Leave crop residue on field to reduce evaporation.

- Diversify livelihoods to avoid depending solely on livestock, which is a risky livelihood strategy.

- Insure animals and crops against death and failures.

- Keep drought-tolerant livestock, like camels.

- Conduct organized grazing patterns to reduce overgrazing and enable regeneration grazing lands.

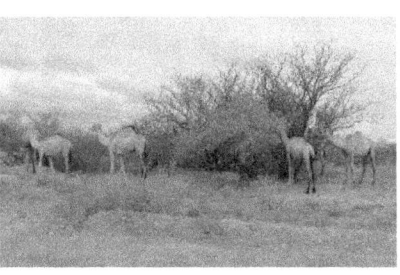

- Sell animals through offtake programme

- Initiate village support systems, like loans and saving schemes.

- Make ghee, dried meat, and fodder for dry season.

- Slaughter old or weak livestock for consumption.

- Reduce the number of meals per day.

- Split household by sending some children to relatives.

- Link children to the school feeding programmes.

- Seek relief assistance, including food, water, or cash transfers from government and humanitarian agencies if there is possibility of being overwhelmed.

- For those in urban areas, store water and power to avoid rationing disruptions.

Chapter 7

EARTHQUAKES AND BUILDING SAFETY

The cases of building failures and consequent collapse of structures in Kenya, and more specifically urban areas, has reached an alarming state in the past few years.

In one of the worst incidents in May 2016, a seven-storey building which was dangerously constructed on the riparian area collapsed killing 51 people in Huruma Estate, Nairobi.

In 2015 alone, seventeen buildings collapsed, including a case in Roysambu along Thika Road where seven people died.

Earlier in December 2014, more than 12 people died after two multi-storey residential buildings that were partly occupied and still under construction collapsed in Kaloleni and Huruma estates in Nairobi.

These cases exemplifies the many instances that tenants have been subjected to dangerous occupancy, resulting into loss of lives and property worth millions of shillings.

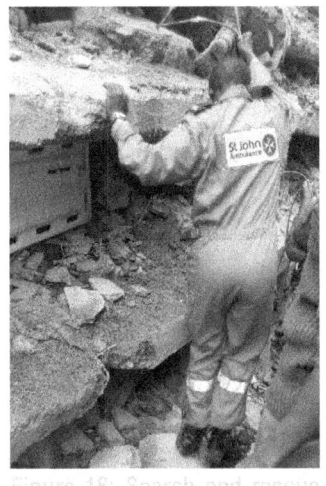

Figure 18: Search and rescue teams in desperate attempts to recover victims of a collapsed seven-storey building in Nairobi's Huruma Estate.

A number of reasons have been cited to explain why these buildings collapsed, including poor workmanship, use of substandard materials, cost-cutting by contractors and a multitude of other reasons.

During a forum in Nairobi in June 2015 on *measures to curb the collapsing of buildings* in the country, the government revealed that 52 per cent of the structures in Nairobi have defects, and should either be restructured or demolished.

These findings confirmed an earlier report by *Questworks* in 2014, which discovered that 3 out of 4 buildings in Nairobi would be damaged in the event of a major earthquake.

The study found that the quality of construction work is poor across Nairobi, but was more alarming in less affluent estates. The findings also revealed that contractors who steal cement and use less steel are to blame for most of the weaknesses.

The unfortunate characteristic in almost all occasions of building collapse is that there has been obvious warning signs of collapse, but tenants perilously ignore these telltale signs.

But even thereafter, nothing tangible is undertaken in the wake of such disasters, besides the occasional tough talk by authorities, which fizzles out as soon as the debris is cleared and the victims buried.

It is therefore imperative that everyone learns how to determine a dangerous structure and ways of staying safe.

7.1 Red Flags of Imminent Building Collapse

Many occupied buildings in Kenya are not approved by the authorities, or the developers change the approved designs to accommodate their own selfish interests, endangering the lives of tenants.

So before you get buried in the debris, here are the telltale signs of imminent structural collapse you need to worry about and vacate:

- Buildings constructed on waterway or riparian area.

- Structural cracks, mostly leading to foundation.

- Large separation of bricks and badly slanting floors.

- Water seeping from walls and ever-flooded basement.

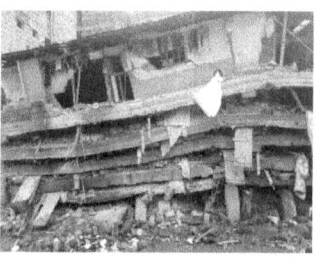

Figure 19: Site of a collapsed building in Huruma, Nairobi.

- Weird crack sounds, especially during strong winds.

- Flats that go beyond four flours without an elevator.

- Flats partly occupied and upper floors under construction.

Make sure you consult an expert in case you notice your building has most of these telltale signs. Better be safe than sorry!

7.2 Escaping from a Collapsing Building

Poor workmanship and use of substandard materials have been cited as the main reason for collapsing buildings in Kenya.

Likewise, an act of terrorism, earthquake, flooding or landslides can cause even a brand new, sound building to collapse.

Regardless of what causes the collapse, there are interrelated ways to survive and escape death or severe injury.

Usually, the collapse occurs very quickly, leaving you with a few seconds for escape and quick action.

If you are escaping from a building with an elevator, do not use the elevator, because the elevator is a death trap! If the building were to collapse, the elevator could plummet off its pulley system, most likely to your death.

You will be much safer, and possibly live longer, using the stairs to escape.

However, when you notice that the wall is caving in and you cannot get out in time, position yourself next to a sturdy piece of furniture such as heavy desk, sofa, or large overstuffed armchair, lying on the floor in fetal position.

The furniture will be able to support a collapsing wall and create a space adjacent to it where you will be relatively safe (this area is known as the triangle of life). In this position, you may get injured, but chances are that you will come out of the wreckage alive.

For safety sake, do not get under any furniture, as was earlier suggested in outdated "duck and cover" tactic, which has glaring illogicalities. Its deficient justification was that falling debris would fall off the furniture, when in reality, the collapsing walls or ceiling would come straight down, crushing the people hiding under these items to death.

Once the building has finished collapsing and there is no more movement, then it is time to carefully assess the situation.

If you find that you are having trouble breathing, cup your hands over your nose and mouth and breathe into them.

If you have an electronic device of any kind with a cellular signal, use it. If not, stay where you are and call loudly for help.

However, do not waste all of your energy screaming after you see that nobody is coming anytime soon. Instead, conserve your energy and use it only when you hear a rescue party is near.

Remaining calm throughout the building collapse is easier said than done, and one of the biggest mistakes that people do is to scream and shout for hours only to quickly become exhausted.

Not only does screaming raise your heart rate and breathing, but you will be inhaling more toxic fumes, dust particles, and other micro debris that can quickly have a negative effect on your lungs and airways.

7.3 | Earthquake Safety

E arthquakes have never occurred in the history of Kenya. However, earth tremors have been witnessed across the country.

In many instances, earthquake or tremor warnings are issued well in advance, giving time for vulnerable populations to evacuate.

Follow the following safety guidelines:

- Do not ignore such warnings, even if they are false alarms.

- Beware of other hazards triggered by earthquakes e.g. damage to buildings, highways, and other structures.

- Never flee outside a building when an earthquake strikes. You may get injured or killed by falling debris or glass. Wait until the shaking has stopped.

- To stay safe, get next to a sturdy piece of furniture so that if a wall falls, it will create a "triangle of life" space in which you can survive if you lie in fetal position.

- Use your hands and arms to protect the vital organs such as head and chest from falling objects.

- Slowly and carefully leave the building to a designated assembly point.

- Avoid stopping near, or under buildings, trees, overpasses, and utility wires. They can fall onto you.

- Avoid driving on roads, bridges, or ramps that might have been damaged by the earthquake.

TRANSPORTATION SAFETY

When it comes to safety on the roads, Kenyans have perfected the art of blaming one another, with the police blaming civilians for being hard-headed and civilians blaming police for being pathologically corrupt.

After every road accident, the blame game escalates, then fizzles out as soon as the bereaved bury their dead. But it does not take long before more Kenyans die on the roads.

Kenyans then take to social media to complain, and from the conversation you could pick that almost everyone is knowledgeable and love talking about road safety, but are very slow in implementing or observing road safety measures that can reduce road carnage.

As a result, about 3,000 road deaths occur every year in Kenya. A recent report by transport safety authority indicates that 2,965 people died from road crash in 2016, which is a marginal drop of three percent compared to 3,057 in 2015.

Pedestrians, motorcyclists and their pillion passengers account for more than half of all road fatalities, but enforcing safety laws on this category is a challenge, and often met with hostility.

The Northern Corridor, which traverses across 11 counties is a significant contributor to road crashes, especially at the notorious accident blackspots.

Road users are likely to die on Fridays and weekends, as more than half of the road deaths occur on these days. Some of the factors leading to these fatalities include drink-driving, drink-walking, drink-riding and motorists using unfamiliar roads.

Other risky behaviors to blame for the rising toll on Kenyan roads include speeding and dangerous overtaking. Overlapping matatus and boda bodas who violate traffic regulations also contribute to road deaths.

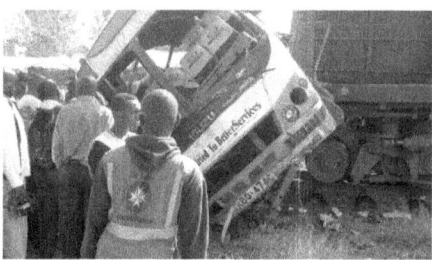

Figure 20: 13 passengers lost their lives after a train rammed into a matatu. The accident was blamed on the carelessness of the driver

The traffic deaths are a major concern and needs urgent action to achieve the ambitious road safety targets (3.6 & 11.2) reflected in the Sustainable Development Goals (SDG) and the UN Decade of Action for Road Safety 2011-2020.

SDG target 3.6 aims to reduce global road deaths and injuries by 50% by 2020 and SDG target 11.2 aims to provide access to safe, affordable, and accessible transport for all by 2030.

The traffic crashes also have enormous consequences to the country, with World Bank estimating the economic cost at 5.6% of the GDP (about 300 billion Kenya shillings) annually.

8.1   Post-crash Care (First Aid)

The rising cases of road deaths is becoming a big concern in the country.

But of more concern is that, more than half of these road deaths are as a result of poor handling and incorrect first aid given by first responders; accounting for about 57 per cent of victims of road accidents according to St John Ambulance.

For this reason, if a responder is not trained on first aid, the best help they can give to an accident victim is to call for an ambulance or police.

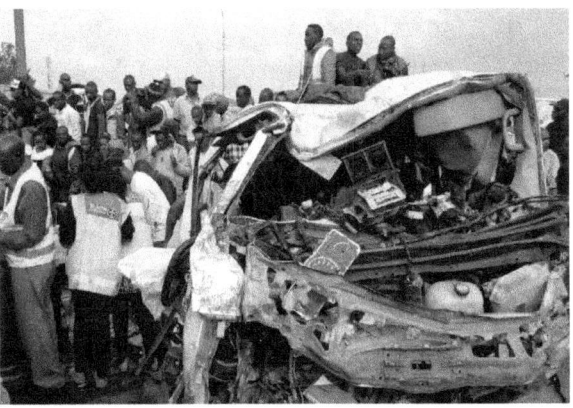

These are the hotlines to call: St John Ambulance 0721-225285, Red Cross 0700-395395, and Police 999/112.

When calling, it is not guaranteed that an ambulance will be available, but the caller can be given vital first aid instructions over the phone on how to stabilize the casualties as they wait for alternative help.

Be keen to listen to the instructions even though the situation may be tense, as giving wrong or doubtful fast aid treatment may only worsen the survivor's chance of living.

Nonetheless, your first action at an accident scene should be to assess for any hazard such as being run over by oncoming motorist, dangerously hanging vehicle or explosive chemicals like petrol.

You can use reflective lifesavers or modified twigs, to alert oncoming motorists of the impending danger.

Always remember to wear gloves or modify polythene to protect yourself from cross-infection by the casualty's blood and other body fluids.

While giving care, wailing survivors, who are not seriously injured, should not detract your attention from caring first for critical victims, who in most occasions are silent or unconscious.

This is because unconscious accident victims have not as much of time to stay alive compared to others. They may be having blocked airway, which could easily lead to death after four minutes if someone does not offer simple intervention like opening their airway by tilting the head upwards.

In case of a bleeding wound, use gloved hand or casualty's hand to apply pressure on the wound area to stop blood loss, then cover the injured area with a clean clothing or bandage.

Do not dislodge any embedded object on a wound, as this may open closed blood vessels, then trigger profuse bleeding. As an alternative, protect the object in place with bulky dressings before bandaging.

But in a worst-case-scenario, like spinal injury, the casualty should not be moved at all, unless they are exposed to further dangers, such as fire or being run over by oncoming motorists.

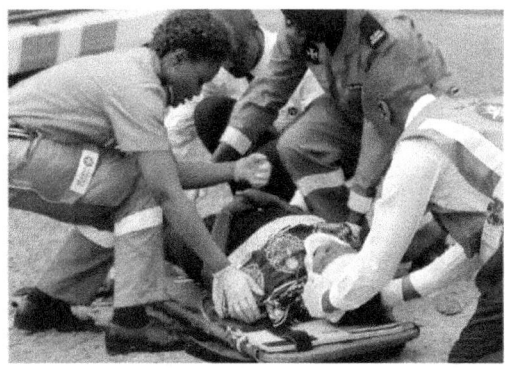

Instead, hold the victim's neck area in the position you find it until paramedics arrive with spinal stabilization equipment.

When you finish the rescue operations, it is important to clear any used first aid materials off the scene and dispose appropriately to avoid infection from blood and other body fluids.

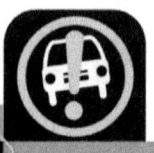

8.2 | Preventing Road Accidents

Accidents just take a second to happen but suffering takes a lifetime.

Some of the most dangerous habits, often leading to fatal road accidents and need to be addressed include drunk driving, speeding, dangerous overtaking, and distractions.

By actively avoiding these four main causes of road deaths, drivers really can make it possible to lower the road toll.

Motorists need to drive at a speed that allows them to spot hazards and react accordingly.

Moreover, the temptation of driving, riding or walking on the road under influence of alcohol should be remote in a everyone's thought.

The drivers should also avoid dangerous overtaking and distracted driving activities such as using a cell phone, sleeping on the wheel, stealing a quick glance at an attractive pedestrian, and eating. Similar distractions should be avoided by pedestrians.

Night driving is also one of the most dangerous activities to do. Of all fatal car accidents, at least 49-percent occur at night, despite there being fewer drivers on the road.

This is partly because, dosing and drunk drivers are more likely to be on the road at night.

The most obvious way to avoid the dangers inherent to night driving is to simply not drive at night, or avoid driving at times when you would usually be asleep.

Feeling tired when you are driving is an early warning sign that you will fall asleep at the wheel. Consequences can be fatal if you choose to ignore this tell-tale sign.

In addition, do not drive on free gear to save on fuel. It's difficult to re-engage brakes or gears when free-wheeling downhill leading to fatal accidents.

Finally, ensure that your car is regularly checked and maintained.

8.3 Accident Blackspots

There are over 200 accident black spots identified along major highways across the country. This is according to data from the traffic police department and Safe Way Right way, a road safety non-governmental organization.

Rift Valley has the greatest number, with more than 12 black spots, while North Eastern has the least at five. Motorists need to be careful while traveling along these spots.

Nairobi Region

In Nairobi County, Mombasa Road and Thika Superhighway are the top killers. Other killer roads are Eastern Bypass, Kangundo Road, and Northern Bypass. On Waiyaki Way, the area near Kangemi flyover is a black spot. Users of Jogoo Road are at the greatest risk at Maziwa Stage.

According to the National Transport and Safety Authority, over 70 per cent of Nairobi's accident fatalities are pedestrians.

Eastern region

In Eastern Region, Nithi Bridge along the Meru - Embu road is one of the most notorious spots for accidents. Other listed blackspots are along Mombasa Road at Lukenya, Kapiti Slopes, and Mazeras. Kemco Turbo section also has a sharp bend and tall vegetation that compromise on visibility.

Coast region

In the Coast Region, most accidents occur at Kibarani – Changamwe stretch, Mtongwe Junction on Lunga Lunga-Likoni road, Tsavo-Maungu-Voi section, Wundanyi-Mwatate, Malindi at Jiwe Tanga and several other stretches of the road.

Western region

In Western, one is likely to die in a road crash on the Mbale-Vihiga road, Kakamega-Chavakali road, Kakamega-Webuye, Kakamega –Ilesi-Kisumu road, and Matayos among other notorious sections.

Nyanza region

Black spots in Nyanza include Awasi-Ahero Road, Kiboswa-Kisumu Road, Daraja Mbili-Bondo Junction, Oyugis-Katitu Road and Migori-Kakrao Road.

Other notorious spots are Gucha Bridge, Migori Township, Kisii Township Main Road, Mwembe Area Kisii Town and Kisii Daraja Mbili.

Central region

In Central Kenya, the Kiganjo-Narumoru road, Kibirigwi to Sagana, Limuru to Uplands and the Kiriani-Muranga roads are some of the worst killer spots in the region.

Rift Valley region

The Naivasha-Nakuru highway is also a dangerous stretch of road to be on the lookout for especially at the Kinungi junction, Gilgil junction and Maili Mbili in Naivasha.

Drivers should also be wary while driving along the Nakuru-Timboroa-Burnt forest area, the Salgaa-Molo stretch, Kericho - Kaitui section, Eldama Ravine-Makutano Junction, Timboroa - Burnt Forest section, Chepsir - Kipkelion Junction and the Mai Mahiu-Narok slopes.

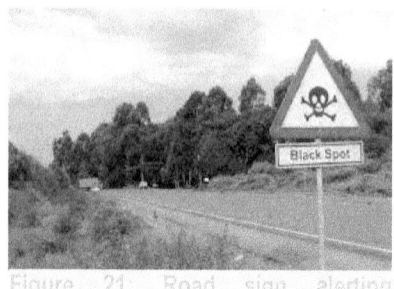

Figure 21: Road sign alerting motorists of a blackspot at Sachangwan along Nakuru-Eldoret Highway

Northern Region

North Eastern has the fewest spots, perhaps because of the poor road network in the region. Some of the black spots in the area are Garissa Madogo-KBC Station, Modogashe-Habaswein, and Bangale-Hola Road.

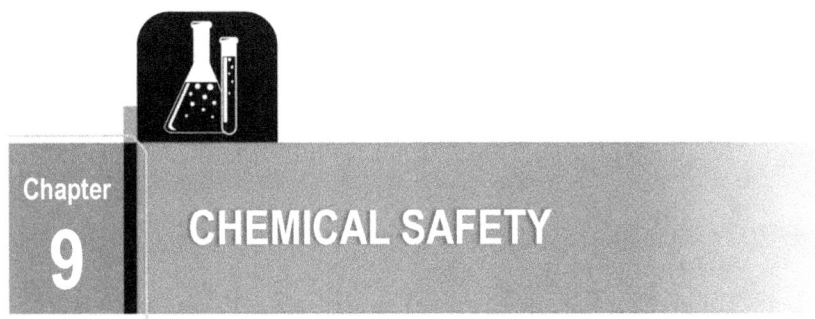

CHEMICAL SAFETY

C hemical spillage has in the past affected Nairobi's Juakali area where artisans handling scrap metals and waste containers are exposed to toxic gases and other chemicals.

But more inexcusable is that populations are still living on top of the petroleum pipeline passing through Sinai area in Nairobi, despite the fact that more than 120 people lost their lives on the same spot when underground oil tunnel exploded.

Some incidents of spillage are also witnessed during storage and transportation of fuels and other hazardous materials by tankers.

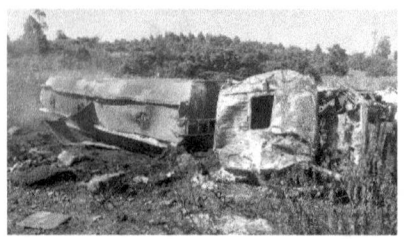

Figure 22: Petroleum tanker involved in an accident bursts into flames after residents attempted to syphon fuel at Kaitui in Kericho

These mostly occurs near black spot areas along the northern corridor, such as Sachangwan and Salgaa.

Radiation and nuclear emergencies though not common, has got the potentiality to contaminate large territories and affect the living conditions of communities.

Kenya is currently strengthening national arrangements for response to radiological and nuclear emergencies and improve compliance with international standards.

9.1 Actions during Toxic Spills

If you find yourself at a site of a toxic spill:

↪ Move quickly into an area with clean air in order to minimize exposure to the gas and fumes.

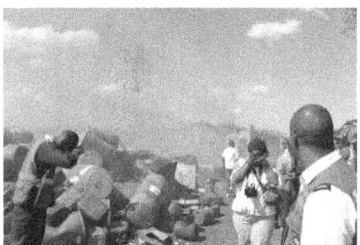

Figure 23: Toxic smoke from burning chemicals at Nairobi's Juakali area

↪ Once you are safely out of the area of the toxic leak, call for emergency services and wait for help to arrive.

↪ Always stay upwind.

↪ Eliminate ignition sources like smoking or lighting a match.

↪ Soak any fabric in urine or water and hold it up to your nose as a mask. Urine crystallizes the gas.

↪ Cut the clothes off that may have been exposed to the gas or fumes.

↪ Clean your body thoroughly with a lot of water and soap.

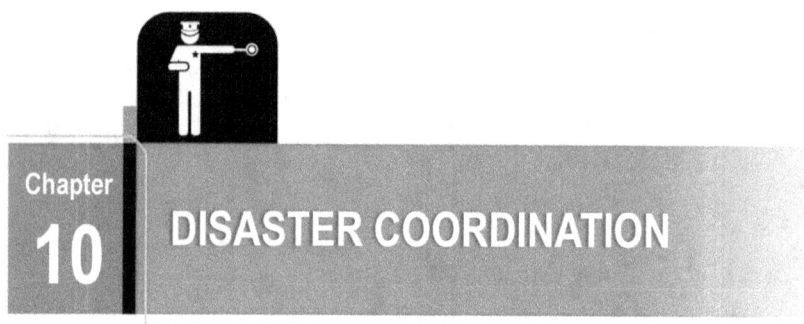

DISASTER COORDINATION

Response to disasters can be chaotic, with arguments and jostling between various agencies over who is in charge.

For instance, when Al-Shabaab gunmen killed 67 people during a four-day siege at Nairobi's Westgate Mall in 2013, confusion played out between police and military.

The soldiers opened friendly fire upon police officers from the elite Recce Squad, perhaps because they were mistaken for terrorists. This triggered an ugly exchange of words between the military and police.

Besides both teams being trained exhaustively on Incident Management System (IMS), which is an organized inter-agency approach to seamlessly work together in managing disasters, it was ignored with deadly consequences.

Instead, there was a tussle over command and control of the operation, creating a tributary tragedy.

The misunderstanding between different agencies involved in the operation pointed to a bigger problem of power struggle which always jeopardise coordination at disaster sites.

To avoid such mix-ups playing out, it's vital that all responders, adhere to Incident Management System, which lays down protocols for handling both the initial incident and its aftermath.

The system was initiated by America after the confusions of the 9/11 attacks, and has been adopted globally as an efficient multi-agency coordination approach during disasters of mass-casualty in nature.

The system provides flexible, but standardized approach for managing incidents.

The protocols range from setting up incident command centres to handling unrelenting media inquiries as well as managing donations and psychosocial support.

These protocols, at times referred to as Incident Command System (ICS), can help reduce crisis chaos, increase first responder efficiency and assist the emotional recovery of victims and families.

The protocols and action plans should not be weighed down by bureaucracy or inter-agency infighting.

They also need to be kept fairly simple for quick understanding by lay persons supporting the expert rescuers.

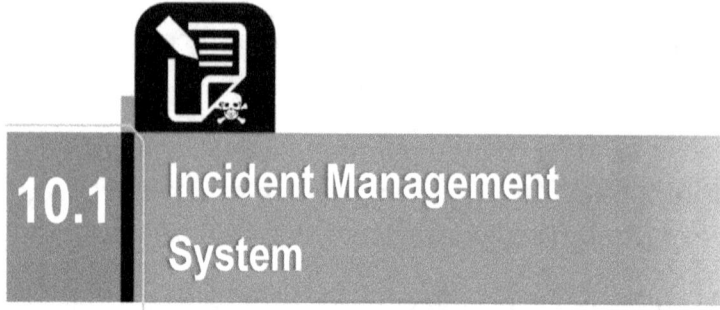

10.1   Incident Management System

The incident management system provides guiding principles to enable agencies with different functional responsibilities work together, synergizing their resources and structure to improve efficiency.

As they join in the rescue effort, each agency seamlessly fits in their personnel, equipment and communications to operate within a common organizational structure.

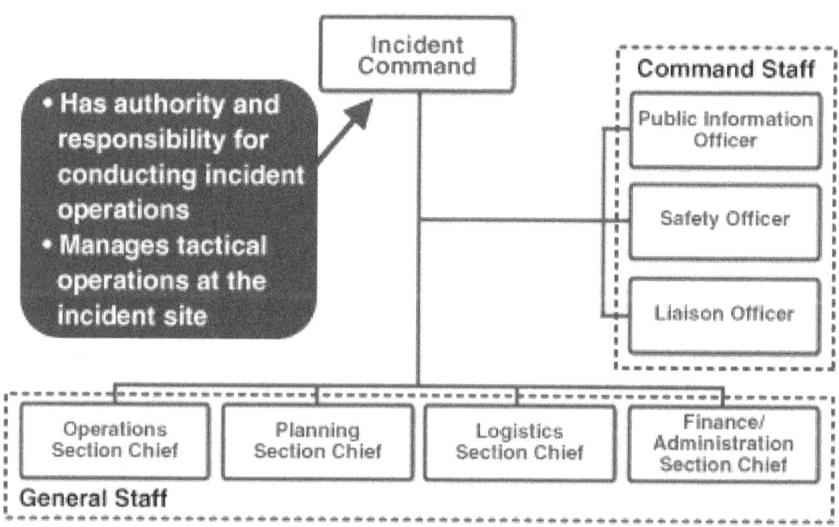

Figure 24 : Incident Management Teams (SOURCE:FEMA)

The structure usually consists of command staff managing the public information, safety and liaison functions.

Other teams handle the operations, planning, logistics, finance and administration functions as highlighted below:

Operations: responsible for all tactical activities focused on reducing the immediate hazard, saving lives and property, establishing situational control, and restoring normal operations.

Planning: responsible for gathering, analyzing, foretelling and giving out of operational information as well as documentation of Incident Action Plan.

Logistics: Responsible for providing facilities, food services, security, transportation, supplies, equipment maintenance and fuel.

Finance and Administration: Responsible for financial considerations including, contracting, cost analysis, compensation and claims.

10.2 | Incident Action Plans

The incident action plan defines objectives and tactics needed in managing an incident during an operational period.

Each incident, may have different plan of action. Nonetheless, these are some of the vital plans to put in place during a disaster: Command center, safety, site access, medical services, public information (communications), decontamination, search and rescue, body management, mental health (psychosocial support), logistics and donations.

Command Centre

- ⮐ At the onset of any incident, determine the incident commander first. Do not spend too much time on this, as it's not the best time to bicker over who is in charge.

- ⮐ The first responder at scene can take charge, but may seamlessly transfer command to a person with primary authority for overall command, control and coordination of the incident like police.

- ⮐ Locate the incident command centre with reasonably close proximity to the incident.

- ⮐ Make sure there is enough room for parking, a sheltered area for distributing food and temporarily storing donations, and meet the sanitary needs of the emergency personnel.

- Consider a separate location for the media; roped off with access allowed only for credentialed journalists.

- On arrival at incident scene, all responders need to identify and report to the incident commander, who has overall responsibility for managing objectives, strategies, and action plans.

- Fence off the command centre to allow control of onlooker access to the centre.

Safety

In any disaster situation it is essential that you take precautions to ensure your own safety and the safety of others. Potential dangers may result from:

- Unsafe scene like oncoming traffic or fallen power lines in a road accident.

- The presence of smoke, fire or poisonous fumes.

- Secondary collapse, falling debris or flying objects.

- Secondary attack or explosion by terrorists.

- Acts of aggression or violent mobs.

- Anxious onlookers placing themselves and others at risk of injury.

- Exposure to blood, vomit and other body fluids.

- Back, neck or shoulder injuries sustained when moving objects.

The following are some of the key steps that a first responder carefully does to protect themselves and others from dangers:

- Always assess and size-up the scene for any potential dangers and ensure the area is safe even before contact with survivors.

- Use protective gears, such as wearing helmet, visibility jacket, boots and gloves, to protect yourself from falling objects or cross-infection with blood and other body fluids.

- Do not unnecessarily move casualty or heavy objects.

- Observe and manage onlookers.

- Seek professional counselling and debriefing, if exposed to horrifying scenes.

Site Access

- Ensure adequate access to the scene is maintained at all times.

- Create a safe perimeter around the incident. An area where emergency personnel can be relatively safe.

- Be prepared for an onslaught of medical, police, fire, media and civilians to approach the incident area.

- The command centre may consider implementing a day-pass accreditation procedure to restrict access to the site to authorized personnel only.

- Site access issues can be reduced by implementing a 12hr on/12hr off schedule for first responders. Briefings before each shift and debriefings after each shift should be mandatory.

Medical Services

There are three phases of medical services at an emergency site i.e. triage, onsite stabilization, and transportation.

(a) Triage

In most mass casualty situations, the number of patients usually exceed the number of rescuers, ambulances and medical facilities.

Triaging is therefore done to separate out minor injuries, and reduce the urgent burden on medical facilities.

Create a victim triage area nearby the incident and secondary triage area for ambulance pickup. Depending on the size and type of the crisis, more than one area may be required.

During triage, four aspects are evaluated: (1) Ability to walk, (2) respirations, (3) blood circulation, and (5) mental status. The assessment takes less than 30 seconds for each victim.

Based on assessment, casualties are placed into one of the following categories:

- Acute condition (*Red tag*) - Mostly unconscious, with air circulation present after positioning the airway. Require immediate evacuation.

- Serious condition (*Yellow tag*). These victims generally cannot walk, but can follow basic instructions, such as raising the arms. Their evacuation can be delayed.

- Walking wounded (*Green tag*) - Minor conditions, requiring medical attention but is able to walk.

- Deceased (***Black tag***) - No ventilations present after the airway is opened. Presenting signs of obvious death including: decomposition, decapitation (beheading), dependent levity (accumulation of fluid on one lower side of body), and rigor mortis (stiffness of the body).

When you begin triaging victims:

- Instruct the patients who can walk to go to a predetermine treatment area, and tag them green.

- Clear them from the area so that you can remain with more serious injured victims to triage.

- Next, ask for victims who can hear you to carry their hands or legs, and tag them yellow.

- Proceed to the remaining victims, tagging them either red or black depending on your assessment.

- During assessment, check for breathing first. If breathing is not present, reposition the airway. If they are still not breathing, triage as dead.

- Check respiratory rate if opening airway results in breathing. If the victim is breathing more than 30 times per minute, triage as immediate (red tag).If breathing is less than 30 times per minute, check for radial pulse at the wrist.

- If radial pulse is present, check for mental status, and tag immediate (red tag) if the victim cannot follow simple instructions. If the patient can follow simple instructions, tag as delayed (yellow tag).

If a victim is triaged as immediate (red tag), repositioning the airway and controlling severe bleeding are the only initial treatments performed before moving on to the next victim.

Triage categories are updated by reassessing and retagging appropriately.

It is also important that a quick but reliable patient registration process is implemented to avoid delays in patient care or confusion over patient location.

(b) Onsite Treatment

Upon reaching the victim, perform initial assessment on a casualty, which include checking for life-threatening conditions such as responsiveness, airway, breathing, and severe bleeding.

Thereafter, a secondary assessment is done to find out the mechanism of injury or nature of illness as well as medical history of the victim.

Continuously monitor the breathing, pulse, and body temperature of the casualty and not any changes.

Because of the risk of aggravating a spine injury, do not move the victim to perform assessment except when the casualty faces immediate danger like fire or explosion.

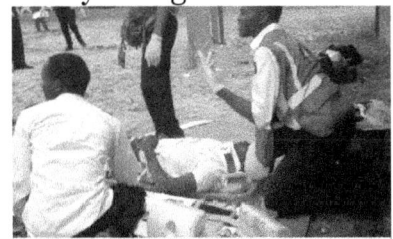

Figure 25; Figure 12 2: Stabilizing victim of spine injury on the scene.

Provide Basic Life Support treatment (*details in Part II: Emergency Medical Care*), and transportation to appropriate hospital with required facilities.

You may consider calling the hospital first to determine availability of critical care facilities if required.

(c) Transportation to Hospital

Evacuation using ambulances is useful in a disaster to:

- ⊃ Decompress the disaster area;
- ⊃ Improve care for most critical casualties by removal to off-site medical facilities; and
- ⊃ Provide specialized care for specific casualties, such as those with burns and crush injuries

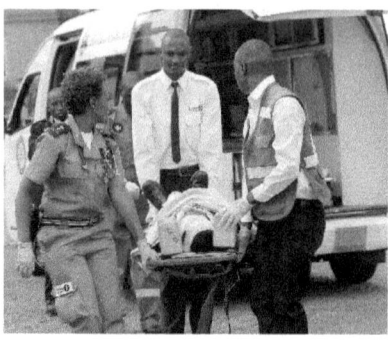

Figure 26: Medics preparing to load a patient in an ambulance for transportation to hospital

Sometimes medical evacuation could be delayed or deferred e.g. contaminated casualties, casualties with transmissible diseases, and unstable casualties.

Decontamination

Any disaster victim exposed to chemical, radioactive or other contaminated materials is transported by properly protected personnel to the decontamination area prior to treatment.

If exposed to hazardous materials, remove or cut the clothes off that may have been exposed to the toxic spill. Thereafter, clean your body thoroughly with a lot of water and soap.

Government Chemist, KDF HAZMAT team, or Radiation Protection Board may be required to decontaminate Chemical, Biological, Radiological and Nuclear materials.

Search and Rescue

Search and rescue involves the location, rescue (extrication), and initial medical stabilization of victims trapped in confined spaces.

Building collapse is most often the cause of victims being trapped, but victims may also be trapped in transportation accidents, mines, drowning, terrorist activities, and hazardous material releases.

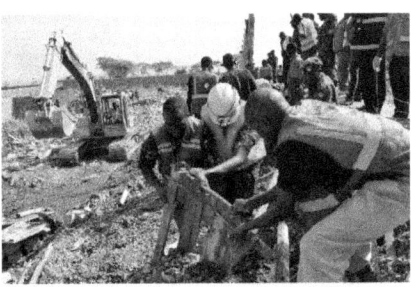

Figure 27: Search and rescue operations ongoing at the site of a collapsed building in Mlolongo, Machakos County

Fire departments have specialized extrication equipment used in the search and rescue operations. They are assisted by trained responders.

If overwhelmed, other heavy excavation machines and expertise may be sourced from the military or road contractors.

In case of hazardous materials, the expertise and equipment of the Government Chemist or military HAZMAT team may be required. Radiation Protection Board may also be required to mitigate and decontaminate Radiological and Nuclear materials.

Body Management

Body recovery is done spontaneously by a large number of individuals, including: Surviving community members, volunteers (St. John ambulance, Kenya Red Cross Societies, etc.), search and rescue teams, military, or police.

Recovery of bodies is least prioritized so as not interrupt other interventions aimed at helping survivors.

Bodies are placed in body bags, or alternatively in plastic sheets, bed sheets, or other locally available material.

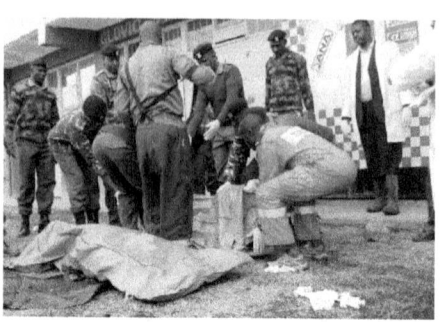

Figure 28: Labeling of bodies at the site of a plane crash in Utawala, Nairobi.

Police vehicles or hearse is used to transport bodies to the mortuary. Ambulances CANNOT be used for this purpose, as they are best used to help the living.

Mental Health (Psychosocial Support)

When a rubber band is stretched beyond its resiliency point, it will not resume its normal shape again. It is the same with a person; if they are stretched beyond their emotional resiliency point, they *cannot* recover fully. Therefore;

- Counselling for the victims and families must start immediately.

- Locate a structure such as a school or church to provide briefings and counselling to the victim's families (Family Centre). Twice per day briefings are sufficient.

- Talking to other victims is most effective forms of therapy.

- The Family Centre need to be staffed with clergy and mental health professionals. Support for this centre is often provided by the counselling and humanitarian organizations.

- Set up crisis hotlines to help families and the general public.

- First responders will need at-will access to mental health professionals. Before a breakdown, they need to be able to speak with someone.

Logistics and Donations

- Consider a large, separate, restricted location for donated goods (in addition to the command centre).

- You will require a dedicated team to handle donation logistics and keeping of proper inventory.

- Present a plan of distribution, including an explanation of the timeframes involved.

- Victims and rescue workers need to be fed. Local supermarkets and hotels can be helpful in this regard.

- Send out a call for help to the local business establishments. They can help in ways you may not have considered.

- Dozens of charities pop up in the weeks following an incident; some valid, some fraudulent.

- Be prepared for family squabbles which can interrupt during the distribution of funds to victims' families.

- Most government money is allocated to victims' families for burial expenses.

Communications and Media Briefing

➲ Notify key government officials and agency representatives as soon as possible.

➲ Be prepared to manage multiple of governmental and non-governmental agencies.

➲ Designate a Public Information Officer, with the responsibility of keeping the press up-to-date.

➲ Give at least two briefings at fixed times per day, unless there is significant breaking news.

DEVELOPING A DISASTER PLAN

With myriad of disasters that frequently occur in Kenya, a disaster plan is something necessary for every public institution, and no business should be without.

By creating a disaster plan, you increase the chance that the people around will survive in case a calamity occurs.

A great first step is to recognize the potential dangers that may exist in the surrounding, and work out ways of mitigating and responding to the risks.

The second step is to develop a skeleton plan. Then continue to fill in the blanks over the course of time.

It's a huge project, and can seem overwhelming at the start. But think about it - consider all of the things that could go wrong: fire, flood, workplace violence, terror attack, the death of key employees in a car accident, and the list goes on.

The key is to focus on the likely dangers in your surroundings, and to develop contingency plans for all of those risks.

Part of your plan can include how you will contact each other, and a safe alternative place where you will gather.

This will ensure your everyone knows what to do, where they can go and who they can stay with in the event of an emergency.

An emergency kit is also important, to ensure you will have all of the necessary items for basic survival.

Don't forget the financial plan. Try to have three to five-days-worth of cash to use in the event you can't get to your local bank or ATMs are not available.

Online banking is another way to manage your finances during unsettled times.

Nevertheless, this ten-point list can help you get started with your plan:

1. Organization Commitment

Contingency plan is built on a foundation of organization leadership, commitment and financial support. Without commitment and financial support, it will be difficult to build, update the plan, and maintain resources.

2. Contingency Planning Committee

Appoint an emergency management coordinator and select a group of people who will bring a variety of perspectives on the vulnerabilities to form the contingency planning committee. For instance, you might include high-level managers and representatives from all the departments within your organization.

3. Hazard Mapping

Make a checklist of all hazards, risks and vulnerabilities that are likely to occur in your area and create a list of actions required to combat each hazard. Certain scenarios may be specific to certain businesses units or branches.

4. Tasks and Responsibilities

Divide the action list among committee members according to each member's area of responsibility.

5. Chain of Command

Consider a clear chain of command and authority which is consistent with the order of seniority or succession plan of your organization. If key personnel arc missing, who's in charge? Who makes decisions?

6. Evacuation Plan

Designate marshals, exit routes, assembly points, and equipment (such as fire extinguishers, first aid kits) that may be needed in an emergency. Exit routes should be clearly marked, well lit, wide enough, unobstructed and clear of debris at all times.

7. Disaster Equipment and Supplies

Install fire extinguishers, first aid kit and other emergency items to ensure you have necessary items for basic survival.

8. Emergency Hotlines

It is imperative that your Emergency Planning Committee knows the roles of each disaster support agency and they have an up-dated emergency contact list.

9. Occupant Contacts

Where possible, keep an updated list of the occupant contacts and alternate ways that people can communicate with each other. Include home work and home phone numbers and non-work e-mail addresses. The more ways you have to keep in touch should disaster strike, the better. The list is also used to account for survivors at the assembly point.

10. Training and Testing

Once you have the plan in place, educate your employees about it. Test your plan with mock drills on a regular basis to make sure that everyone in the organization knows how to react.

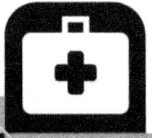

11.1 Emergency Kit

Stock supplies that can save lives!

Stock a first aid kit, fire extinguisher and other survival items like water purifiers and flashlight to ensure you have all of the necessary items for basic survival.

Other items to consider keeping are backup means of charging cellphones.

A well-stocked emergency kit can help you respond effectively to common emergencies.

It is also crucial to check on your emergency kits approximately every six months for expired medications and other outdated requiring replacements.

Keep the items at an easy-to-retrieve locations that are out of the reach of young children. Children old enough to understand the purpose of the kits should know where they are stored.

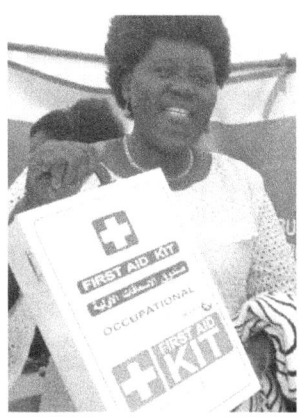

You can purchase these kits from emergency organizations such as St John Ambulance, or at many chemists and supermarkets, or assemble your own.

Figure 29: First Aid Kit

A universal household or travel first aid kit should include these items:

No	Items	Use	Qty
1	Adhesive plaster	Dress small cuts and abrasions	20
2	Adhesive tape	Hold bandage, dressing	1
3	Antihistamine	Relieve stinger allergy	1
4	Burn gel	Reduce pain, infection	3
5	Cotton buds	Cleaning ears, nose	10
6	Crepe bandage	Wrap sprained joints	2
7	Eye pad	Protect injured eye	1
8	Eye wash (normal saline) - 10ml	Clean eyes	3
9	Face Shield	Prevent cross infection	1
10	First-aid leaflet	Simple first aid guide	1
11	Gauze sponge	Clean, cover wounds	3
12	Gloves (pair)	Prevent cross infection	3
13	Instant ice pack	Reduce pain, swelling	1
14	Sanitizer	Clean wounds, hands	1
15	Scissors	Cut dressings, clothing	1
16	tweezer	Stinger removal	1
17	Triangular bandage	Make sling, tourniquet	1
18	Wipes - 10 pack	Wipe dirt	1
19	Sterile wound dressing	Prevent wound infection	3

Medications

Experts debate whether first aid kits should have prescription medications for use in remote locations. One side argues that there is potential for misuse and abuse, while others say this cannot outweigh the victim's wellbeing, health, and need to save a life.

The medications include: activated charcoal (use only if instructed by a Doctor), anti-diarrhea, and aspirin/pain relievers

Emergency Items

- Fire extinguisher

- Bolt cutters

- Emergency hotlines (police, ambulance and fire)

- Flashlight and extra batteries.

- Candles and matches.

- Emergency blanket.

- High-visibility jackets

- Heavy-duty boots

- Barrier tapes

Give your kit a checkup

It is also crucial to check your emergency kit approximately every 6 months to replace expired items.

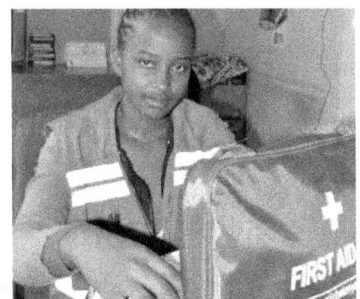

Figure 30: Check kits for outdated items after every six months

11.2 | Emergency Hotlines

With the advent of mobile phones, everyone can access emergency assistance at the touch of a button.

This can only happen if you have the emergency hotlines stored in your phone's contact list.

Some people write emergency contacts in a notebook. But during a crisis, you may not remember where the book was stored.

Equally important, is the need to know situations when to call for emergency help.

An emergency is where health, safety or property is in immediate danger, or there is a crime in progress.

Know
WHEN TO DIAL HOTLINES

➲ When you are in immediate danger or witness a crime in progress.

➲ For a serious injury, medical condition, or any other situation needing urgent attention.

➲ Give information on the number of people affected, precise incident location, events that led to the occurrence, and priority needs.

➲ Be prepared to answer questions and follow instructions from the call-taker, such as step-by-step first aid instructions to help victims.

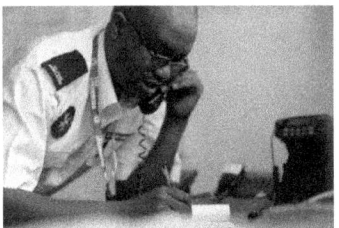

➲ Give important details first, before your phone run out of airtime or battery.

➲ The call-taker may ask about the responsible person for paying, but calling does not impose responsibility on you to pay.

➲ During disasters, wait times may be longer.

➲ Do not dial emergency contacts for non-emergencies or to report a power outage (power outages may be urgent, but phone lines need to be kept open for emergency calls).

WHO TO CONTACT

Service	Organization Name	Hotlines
Ground Ambulance	St John Ambulance	0721225185/0202210000
	E-Plus (Red Cross Ambulance)	0738/0700395395
	AAR Ambulance Service	0725225225
	Avenue Healthcare	0732175150
Air Ambulance	AMREF Flying Doctors	0206992299/000
Firefighting	Nairobi Fire and Rescue Services	0202344599/0771637161
	National Youth Service DRU	0208563521/0208561489
	G4S Fire Services	0711042000/0723786565
	KK Fire Services	0204245000/0730622000
Hospitals	Kenyatta National Hospital	0709854000
Electrical Hazards	Kenya Power	0703070707/0722207999

Security and Disaster Coordination	Kenya Police Service	911/999/112/0202240000
	National Disaster Operations Center	0202212386/0202151053
	Anti-Terrorism Police Unit/CID	0729999988/020512090
	Police Disaster Management Unit	0202188171
Meteorological Emergencies	Kenya Meteorological Services	0203867880/3876957
Forest and Wildlife Emergencies	Kenya Wildlife DRU	0726610508/0206000800
	Kenya Forest DRU	0716277773/0202396440
Hazardous Materials	Military HAZMAT/DRU	0723502413/0202721100
	NEMA	0786101100/0704846019
	Radiation Protection Board	0202689253
	Government Chemist	0202717567/2336300
	Kenya Medical Research Institute	0202722541/2713349
Transportation emergencies	NTSA	0202729200
	Kenya Airport DRU	0206611000/82211
	Kenya Ports DRU	0722208661/2-9
	Kenya Maritime Authority	0721368313/0412131100

*DRU – Disaster Response Unit

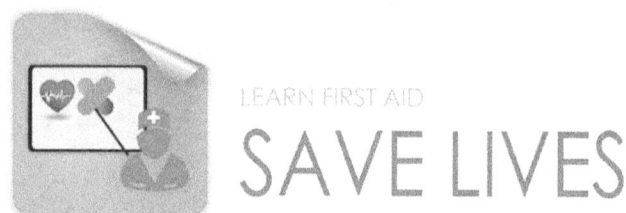

LEARN FIRST AID
SAVE LIVES

PART II: EMERGENCY MEDICAL CARE

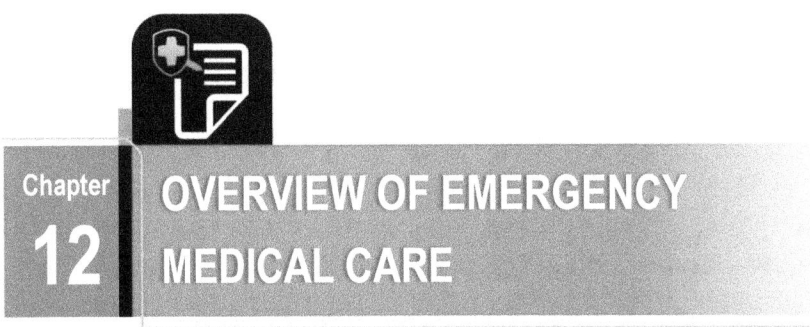

OVERVIEW OF EMERGENCY MEDICAL CARE

In its most basic form, first aid, also referred to as emergency medical care, refers to necessary immediate healthcare that must be administered to save lives and reduce suffering.

The care consists of relatively simple techniques, treatment and support, with an aim to prevent death or worsening of injuries or illnesses.

And in a country where there are many incidents of fire outbreaks, terror attacks and road crashes, the need for everyone to learn first aid skills is vital.

The skills are also crucial for the reason that it takes about 9-30 minutes to get an ambulance, yet some first aid emergencies like chocking can easily lead to death faster, before arrival of an ambulance.

In case of full chocking, there's only four minutes for lifesaving, after which, irreversible brain damage or death is likely.

In such golden moments, it's only basic first aid skills that can make a difference between life and death.

And so, first aid need to be fundamental part of any school or drivers' teaching curriculum.

However, since not everyone has the time or opportunity to learn these skills, it would be beneficial to go through the subsequent sections and acquire a few lifesaving skills that can make the difference.

In these sections, you will learn how to handle urgent first aid emergencies like starting someone's heart, dislodging food when a person is choking, and stopping a fatal bleed.

Other crucial lifesaving skills to learn include handling snake bites, asthma attacks, allergic reactions, and accidental poisonings among others.

You will also know the right way to move an injured person. However, it's always not advisable to move an injured person. But if the person is in immediate danger of fire, flooding, or falling objects, there can be no choice. So you should know the best way to move such a person out of the harm's way.

After learning the first aid skills, it's also vital to have a well-stocked first aid kit with basic necessities needed to treat any minor injuries.

At times, the deaths and gory injuries at disaster scenes can be too traumatizing to handle alone. Hence, psychological first aid skills have also been expounded to help cope with such situations.

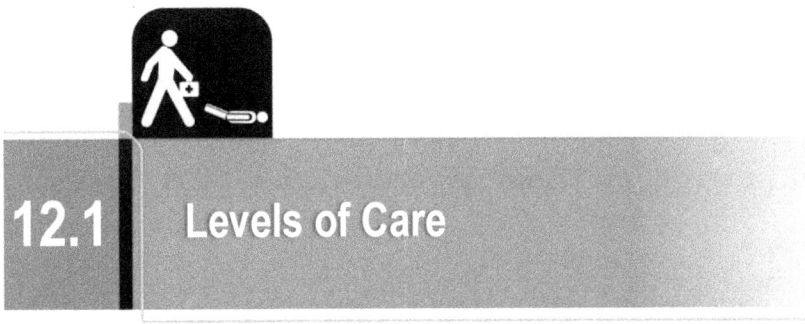

Emergency medical care, is an important and essential part of the healthcare system.

The care is offered in two levels i.e. basic or advanced life support, depending on the caregivers level of training and equipment available for use.

Basic life support is provided by First Aiders, Emergency Medical Responders and Technicians, while Advanced Emergency Medical Technicians (AEMT), Paramedics and critical-care nurses provide advanced life support.

An **Emergency Medical Responder (EMR)**, commonly referred to as **First Responder**, is the first person to arrive at an emergency scene with basic skills necessary in giving emergency care, while waiting for an ambulance to arrive.

Part of the care provided by an EMR include assessing for life-threatening emergency, opening and maintaining airway, ventilating patients, performing resuscitation, controlling bleeding, care for medical emergencies, stabilizing the spine and injured limbs, and assisting with childbirth.

First responders do not give medications, however, some adults may take drugs themselves under doctor's instruction.

In many occasions, a First Responder offers care with limited medical equipment. But they still save lives even without a first aid or trauma kit, though it's essential to have one.

An **Emergency Medical Technician (EMT)**, usually trained for at least 110 hours and works in an ambulance, is more skilled than an EMR and can perform additional care including helping patients with prescribed oral medications such as glucose and activated charcoal.

Advanced Emergency Medical Technicians (AEMT) is more skilled than EMT, and conducts more advanced patient assessment, give intravenous fluids or medications, and perform advanced airway procedures as well as electrocardiogram(ECG) monitoring.

A **Paramedic** has additional education in pathophysiology, physical examination techniques, using heart monitors to assess heart rhythms, and invasive procedures.

First aid is generally not all the treatment a patient needs, but it helps the victim for the short time before advanced care begins. Hence, all acute victims should be referred to hospital.

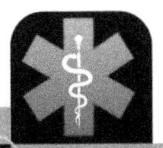

12.2 Phases of Emergency Medical Services (EMS)

Any person professionally involved in patient care needs to know the six phases of emergency medical services. These include:

- ⮑ *Detection* of the emergency by a bystander, then

- ⮑ *Reporting* of the emergency by calling an ambulance hotline, giving clear location of the incident, number of casualties, and potential complications.

- ⮑ *Response* by the First Responder or Ambulance Crew is then activated, as the Ambulance Dispatcher continue to give basic first aid instruction to the bystander to help sustain the life of the casualty.

- ⮑ *On-scene care* is then provided to stabilize the victim after getting quick brief from the first responder. The EMT (paramedics) brief the Dispatcher, and may request for additional ambulances if situation is overwhelming.

- ⮑ *Care during transport* is provided, including ventilations and monitoring the vital signs of life, such as breathing, pulse rate, and blood pressure.

- ⮑ *Definitive care* is finally provided by the hospital attendants after receiving the patient and brief history of care by the ambulance personnel.

Deciding to help

It is not always an easy decision to help victims of an emergency. Many state the following reasons for hesitation:

- *Being upset by the sight of blood, badly burnt skin, vomiting or other conditions.* This is why this book includes stress reduction techniques to help you cope.

- *Not doing the right medical procedure.* However, it's more fatal if you don't do anything at all to help.

- *Thinking someone else will help,* when you should be that "someone else."

- *Catching a disease from the victim.* That is why you need to protect yourself with resuscitation musk, gloves or improvise from polythene bag.

- *Being sued if the victim dies.* But if you offer care as trained, and do everything in the best interest of the casualty, there is no chance of being found legally liable, even if the victim does not recover.

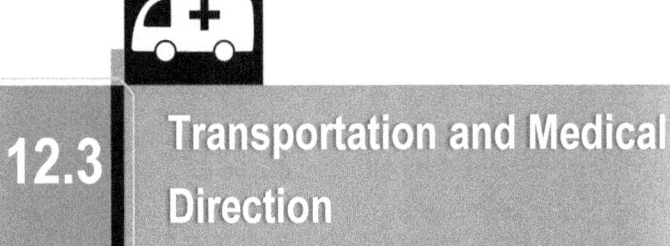

12.3 Transportation and Medical Direction

After providing care and stabilization, some patients may need a properly equipped means of transportation.

The most common means is ground ambulance, though air evacuation is also an option to consider.

Air and ground transport each have advantages and disadvantages; and the decision whether to use air or ground transport should be made on the basis of many factors.

Some of the factors include patient condition, cost, response time, weather, terrain and proximity of a landing site.

The ambulances, whether on ground or airborne, are classified as either basic or advanced life support, depending on the equipment and skill-level of personnel manning it.

Basic life support(BLS) ambulances have equipment and personnel (emergency medical technicians) that provide detailed patient assessment, ventilation, resuscitation, control bleeding, care for medical emergencies, stabilize the spine, and child birth.

They also help patients with prescribed medication and may give oral medication such as activated charcoal.

Advanced Life Support (ALS) ambulances provide intravenous fluids, medications, and advanced airway procedures in addition to everything provided in BLS ambulance.

The ambulances are manned by critical care nurses, clinicians and paramedics, with additional training in pathophysiology, heart rhythm monitoring, and invasive procedures.

In Kenya, the ambulance services are yet to be regulated, and these classifications still do not have a clear-cut differences.

There are also unclassified ambulances such as motorcycle ambulances, and even as donkeys and wheelbarrow ambulance, which are ordinarily uncomfortable, but used as a desperate attempt to save lives in hard-to-reach areas.

Medical Direction

Emergency medics operate sometimes under *medical direction* of an advanced medical practitioner, who give either *offline direction* through policies and protocols, or *online direction* via phone or face-to-face conversation.

Patients are usually stabilized prior to transportation, and care provided throughout the transit to hospital.

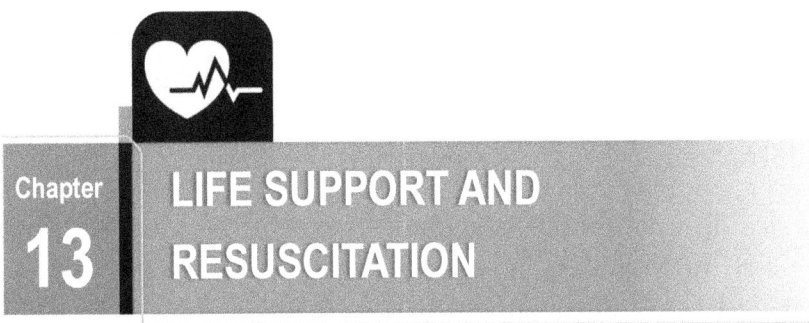

LIFE SUPPORT AND RESUSCITATION

The body is a complex system, consisting of many organs which constantly work to keep it healthy.

Some organs, such as brain, heart and lungs, are so vital that you can't live if they stop. When they fail, a special medical procedure, commonly called life support, is needed to keep you alive until the body is ready to take over again.

Lungs, for instance, can fail in cases of drowning, blood clot, or severe chest injury. Brain likewise can fail due to severe blow to the head or stroke, while the heart can fail as result of sudden cardiac arrest or heart attack.

When most people talk about a person being on life support, they're usually talking about a ventilator, which is a machine that helps someone breathe by pushing air into the lungs.

However, life support refers to a range of methods used to maintain life after the failure of one or more vital organs. For instance, when a person's heart stops, it can be restarted through cardiopulmonary resuscitation (CPR), which keeps oxygenated blood flowing throughout the body. Electric shocks using an automated external defibrillator (AED) may also be used to get the heart beating again.

Other types of basic life support include relief from choking using back-blows and stomach thrusts, and stopping of bleeding by direct compression and elevation above the heart.

Less urgent, though complex forms of life support include dialysis to filter toxins from the blood, and a feeding tube or an intravenous (IV) to give nutrition and water.

Medics are generally certified to perform advanced life support procedures; however, basic life support can be provided by family, friends or Good Samaritans before an ambulance arrives.

On arrival at an emergency scene, the first step is to size up the scene to determine if the situation is safe, number of patients involved, and mechanism of injury or nature of illness; gather an initial impression; and call for additional resources including equipment and ambulance as needed.

After completing the scene size-up and determining that it is safe to approach the patient, you need to conduct primary assessment of the patient, which include determining level of responsiveness, breathing and circulation.

In unresponsive casualty, you may need to open the airway first by lifting the chin, then check for breathing. If breathing is absent you need to call for an ambulance before proceeding with further care.

13.1 Scene Size-up

Scene size-up entails quickly looking at the entire scene to find out if there are any threats that may cause injury to you, other rescuers, bystanders or casualties.

It's made up of 5 parts:
- Evaluating scene safety.
- Determining the total of patients and need for additional resources
- Precautions for cross-infection.
- Determining the mechanism of injury

Scene safety

Scene safety is an assessment of the entire scene to ensure your well-being and that of other rescuers, the patients, and bystanders. Below are some basic steps and precautions:

- Look for hazards, such as downed power lines, unstable vehicle, possibility of being run over by oncoming motorists and signs of potential violence.

- Make the scene safe, if you cannot make it safe, DO NOT ENTER. If a safe scene becomes unsafe at any point, leave.

- Do not enter active crime scenes until it is under control by law enforcement. Take extra precautions if you suspect crime, or simply call for law enforcement.

- Take precautions for unstable surfaces and slopes.

- If in water, wear flotation device. Open water and moving water rescues require specialized training.

- Avoid toxic substances or low oxygen caused by chemical spill or fire.

- Confined spaces such as caves require self-contained breathing apparatus (SCBA).

- Suspect toxic environment if everyone in the area suffer from similar symptoms.

- Take control at the scene, telling crowds to step back. Introduce yourself to patients and always ask for their consent to any treatment. Be courteous, let patients know you are there to help.

- Maintain an escape route.

Number of patients and need for additional resources

While assessing safety, determine the approximate number of casualties and additional resources required.

In some situations, you may need additional resources, such as law enforcement personnel for security, fire engines to put out inferno or extricate accident victims.

The request for these additional resources should be placed as a soon as the need is determined.

After sizing up the scene, proceed to initial patient assessment to see problems that may exist.

In any emergency, there are low risk of infectious diseases from a victim, and taking steps to avoid being infected greatly reduces the risk.

The infectious pathogens can enter the body through a number of ways, including:

- Coming into contact with infected person's blood or other body fluid.

- Inhaling the infected droplets from air breathed by the victim.

- Pricking by a metal with body fluid from the victim.

- Insect bites.

The following are key precautions to help you avoid coming into contact with the victim's blood or body fluid:

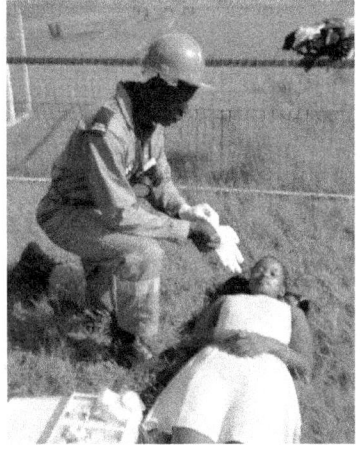

- Use gloves, modify polythene bags, or have the victim dress their own wound.

- If available, use protective equipment such as gown, face mask, goggles or safety boots.

- Wash hands appropriately with soap before and after giving medical care.

- Use resuscitation musk when giving rescue breaths.

- Cover any cuts or scrapes on your skin.

- Do not touch your mouth, nose, or eyes when giving care.

- Be careful not to touch body fluids, or be pierced by anything sharp at emergency scene, such as broken glass or sharp metal.

- Dispose soiled materials appropriately. Soiled clothing should be cleaned with disinfectant or bleach.

- Urgently visit the hospital for post exposure phylaxis (PEP) if you are exposed to a victim's blood.

Procedure for putting on gloves

Step 1: Use fingers of other hand at lower cuff area to pull glove into your thumb, then follow with other fingers.

Step 2: Pull the glove tight. Do not touch your ungloved hand to fingers of gloved hand.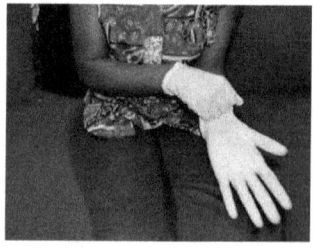

Step 3: Use fingers of gloved hand to pull on other glove.

Procedure for removing contaminated gloves

Step 1: With one hand, grasp your other glove at the wrist or palm, and pull it away from your hand.

Step 2: Remove glove inside out.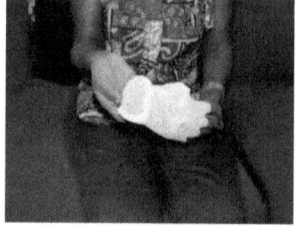

Step 3: Holding the removed glove on gloved hands, insert fingers under the cuff of the remaining glove and pull away inside out.

Mechanism of Injury

Mechanism of injury describes how energy of motion is transferred to an individual resulting in injury. It helps to determine how likely it is that a serious injury has occurred.

A classic example is the motor vehicle crash, in which the extent of damage to the vehicle can be directly related to the extent of injuries the patient may have.

A car crash might be a minor with no damage to the vehicle and no injury to the occupant, or it might be a front-end collision with significant vehicle damage and potentially serious injury to the occupant's head, chest and abdomen.

Falls are another example of how determining the mechanism of injury can be used to estimate the extent of damage to the patient.

The height of the patient's fall, the position in which the patient landed, and the number and kind of objects the patient struck provide valuable information about the patient's potential condition.

For example, a patient who has fallen on an outstretched hand may have a shoulder injury as well as a wrist injury.

Other incidents with potentiality of severe injuries include explosions, violence and burns.

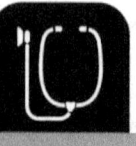

13.2 Initial Patient Assessment

As you approach a patient, form a general impression to determine if he is ill or injured. Also look for any life-threatening problems such as unresponsiveness, obstructed airway, absence of breathing and severe bleeding.

If you find any life threat, it signifies that the victim needs immediate help. Give instant care for the threat as this victim could die if you waste time looking for less-fatal problems like broken bones.

To avoid risk of aggravating paralysis, do not move the victim for assessment except when there is imminent danger like fire.

Checking for Responsiveness

After forming a general impression, begin by speaking to the patient to determine patient's level of responsiveness, using the AVPU scale highlighted below:

Step 1: Alert: the victim is aware of time and place.

Step 2: Voice: the victim is not clearly oriented to time and place, but responds when spoken to.

Step 3: Pain: the victim does not respond when spoken to but feels pain when pinched on the ear.

Step 4: Unresponsive: the victim does not respond to anything.

Opening the Airway

If the airway is not open, there is no breathing, and patient's heart stops beating, unless you open the airway and start breathing for him using resuscitation methods.

Therefore, one of the most important action you need to perform on unresponsive casualty is to open airway by lifting up the chin or jaw bone.

If spinal injury is suspected, never use head-tilt chin-lift maneuver to open the airway. Instead, use jaw-thrust without head-tilt technique to avoid damage to spinal cord.

Follow the following steps to perform head-tilt chin-lift maneuver:

Step 1: Position patient on his back and place the palm of your one hand on the patient's forehead and two fingers of the other hand on the chin, then gently tilt the patient's head backwards.

Step 2: Make sure the patient's mouth is open. Remove visible airway obstruction or loosely fitting dentures.

Where there is risk of spinal injury, such as a patient who is unconscious as a result of a head injury, the airway is opened using jaw-thrust without head-tilt technique, to avoid neck movement. The following steps are performed:

Step 1: Kneel at the top of the casualty's head.

Step 2: Place both hands on both sides of the casualty's lower jaw.

Step 3: Elevate the mandible upwards to lift the tongue and open the airway.

If unresponsive victim's airway is obstructed, you need to clear it through three primary ways: recovery position, suctioning, and finger sweeps.

Victims may be placed in *recovery position*, if you do not suspect spinal injury, to enable the fluids to drain off from the mouth by gravity.

However, for casualties with suspected spinal injury, *suction device* is necessary to clear blood, vomit, and other substances from a victim's airway.

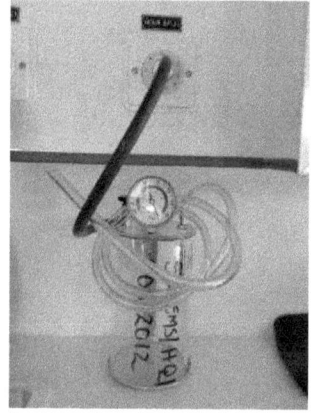

Manual devices develop suction with hand-pumping action. Other devices are powered by battery or pressurized oxygen. Soft rubber bulb syringes are used for suctioning infants.

Be careful not to prolong or suction too deeply to avoid inducing vomiting, bruising, or decrease in oxygen reaching the lungs.

If foreign material is seen in an unresponsive victim's airway, a *finger sweep* may be used to remove it. Blind finger seeps should not be performed if you cannot see the object as it can the object to dislodge further inside.

Checking for Breathing

To check for breathing, lean over with your ear close to the casualty's mouth and nose, and listen to any sound of breathing, feel the warmth of breath, and see the chest rise and fall regularly.

Count the breathing for a minute, or 30 seconds and multiply by two to determine the rate for one minute.

Breathing varies with age: adults breath 12-20 times per minute, while children breath 16-30 times per minute, and infants breath 20-40 times per minute.

Notice any anomaly, for instance, less than 10 breaths per minute in an adult victim is insufficient.

Lack of breathing may be caused by something stuck on the throat, swollen airway tissues due to allergic reaction or neck injury, and by dipping of the victim's own tongue.

If a victim is not breathing, you must immediately give rescue breaths and chest compressions to resuscitate the heart.

If an injured victim is wearing a helmet, it should be removed only if absolutely necessary to care for a life-threatening condition. Removal of a helmet risks worsening of spinal or head injury.

Emergency Helmet Removal

At least two rescuers are required to remove a motorcycle helmet.

- The first rescuer position himself behind the victim's head, open face shield to assess airway, then stabilize the helmet by placing hands on either sides of the helmet with fingers on patient's jaws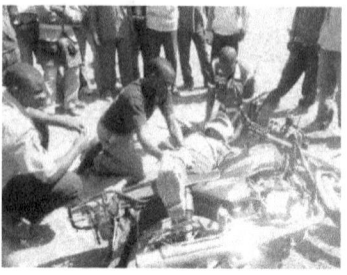

- The second rescuer loosens strap and stabilize the neck area by placing one hand on the lower jaw and the other hand under the neck behind patients head.

- The first rescuer tilts the helmet backward to clear the nose and remove the helmet completely. He then assumes manual stabilization of the head as second rescuer continue with casualty assessment.

Pulse Check

Pulse is an indication of blood circulation to vital body tissues. It also shows the rate at which a heart beats.

As the heart pumps blood through the body, pulsing can be felt in some of the blood vessels close to the skin's surface, such as at the wrist, neck, or upper arm.

To count the pulse rate, simply use your index and middle finger to apply gentle pressure on the artery at the fold on the neck, inside of upper arm, or wrist area. Do not use too much pressure; it may cut off blood flow through the artery. Do not use your thumb to assess pulse – it has a pulse of its own and could be mistaken for a patient's pulse.

Count the number of beats for a minute, or 30 seconds and multiply by two to determine the number of beats per minute (bpm). Begin CPR if pulse cannot be detected for 5-10 seconds.

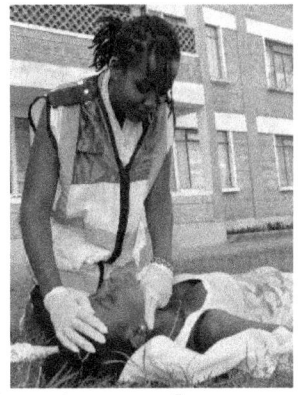

Pulse rate varies with age: Infants (120-160 bpm), children (70-140 bpm), and adults (60-100 bpm)

A pulse oximeter can be used to see if there is enough oxygen in the blood. A reading between 96-100 generally indicate adequate oxygenation, 91-95 suggest mild lack of oxygen in tissues, while a reading below 91 indicates severe deficiency.

Body Sounds and Stethoscope

A stethoscope may be used by emergency medics to listen to body sounds. The device consists of four major parts:

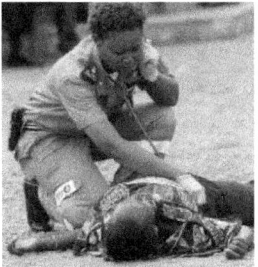

- ⮑ Diaphragm – circular flat part at the end of tubing, used to check sounds, such as breath sounds.
- ⮑ Tubing – should be flexible and about 12-18 inches. Longer tubing decrease sound transmission.
- ⮑ Binaural – metal pieces connecting the earpiece to the tubing.
- ⮑ Earpiece – fit snuggly but comfortably in the ears.

Checking for Severe Bleeding

If the victim is bleeding profusely, vital organs are not receiving enough oxygen to sustain life.

Control any severe bleeding by applying direct pressure with your gloved hands or casualty's hands and give trauma care.

13.3 Cardiopulmonary Resuscitation (CPR)

The body tissues need a nonstop supply of oxygen, and brain cells begin to die, as soon as 4 minutes after oxygen supply is cut off. Within 6 minutes brain damage is likely and death is likely soon after.

Air, containing 16 percent oxygen, is inhaled through the nose, mouth or stoma into the lungs, which absorbs it into blood, then pumps the oxygenated blood to body tissues and organs. Carbon dioxide, a waste product, is picked up and eliminated into the lungs and exhaled.

When this process of breathing is ineffective to an extent the body tissues is not receiving enough oxygen to maintain life, then respiratory emergencies occur.

The cause of respiratory emergencies include obstruction of airway, penetrating chest injury, heart problem, electrical shock, allergy, drug overdose or poisoning.

A victim who is not breathing require rescue breathing to move oxygen into lungs and chest compression to pump oxygenated blood to keep vital organs like brain alive.

This process of rescue breathing combined with chest compressions is called cardiopulmonary resuscitation (CPR), basically trying to do the heart's function of circulating oxygenated blood to vital organs, like brain.

If a victim is unresponsive and not breathing, call for an ambulance first, and then begin CPR. For child victims, call fast after providing 5 cycles of cardiopulmonary resuscitation.

Step-by-step resuscitation technique:

Step 1: Position the victim on his back and tilt the head to open the airway.

Step 2: Position your palm midway between nipples, or just below this line in infants.

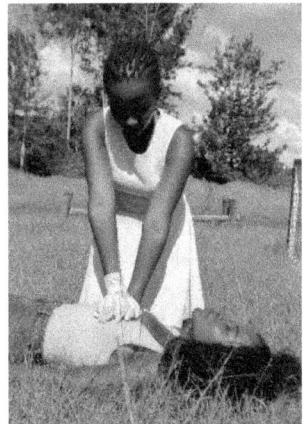

Step 3: Press the chest at a rate slightly faster than a clock's second hand.

Step 4: Using a barrier device to prevent cross-infection, blow air slowly and steadily, rather than too quickly while watching chest rise. Stop each breath when the chest rises to allow the chest to fall between breaths.

If the chest does not rise the airway is blocked and needs care for choking.

Step 5: Alternate 30 chest compressions with 2 rescue breaths for adults.

While giving chest compressions, keep your elbows straight, avoid pressing on the tip of breast bone and minimize time used between rescue breathing and compressions.

In infants, below one year, give 5 Initial breaths followed by 30 chest compressions then resume to 2 breaths.

If you cannot give rescue breaths for unbreathing casualty, you should proceed with chest compressions only. This gives better chance of survival than doing nothing.

Some people breathe through a hole in their neck (stoma). Cup your hands over the victim's mouth and nose then breath normally through the stoma.

Two special problems to avoid during rescue breathing is entry of air in stomach in case of forceful breathing, vomiting and movement of liquids into lungs due to quick breathing, and falling of loose dentures.

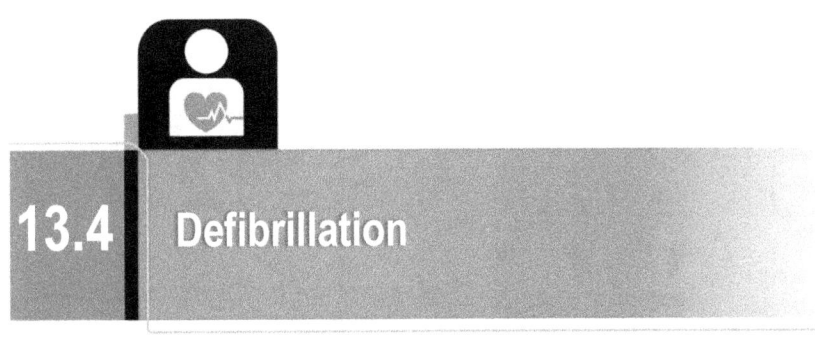

13.4 Defibrillation

An automated external defibrillator (AED) can help get the heart beating normally again after cardiac arrest.

It is connected by cables and pads that automatically monitor the victim's heart and determine whether abnormal rhythm is present for which shock is needed. The unit gives automated instruction on how to use it.

If two rescuers are present, one should begin CPR as the other sets up the device.

Continue CPR until the unit is ready to analyze the victim's heart rhythm, and then stop and follow the unit's instructions.

Procedure for using AED:

Step 1:   Place the AED near the victim's shoulder, and turn it on, then position the victim away from water or metal that can conduct electricity.

Step 2:   Expose the victim's chest, and dry if necessary.

Step 3:   Place the chest pads on victim's chest. They have diagrams to remind you where to position them. (typically, the first pad is placed on right side below the collar bone and the second pad is placed below and to the left of the nipple)

Step 4:   Stand clear of the victim during rhythm analysis.

Step 5: Follow prompts from the AED unit to (a) press the shock button or (b) do not shock but immediately give CPR with the pads remaining in place, starting with the chest compressions.

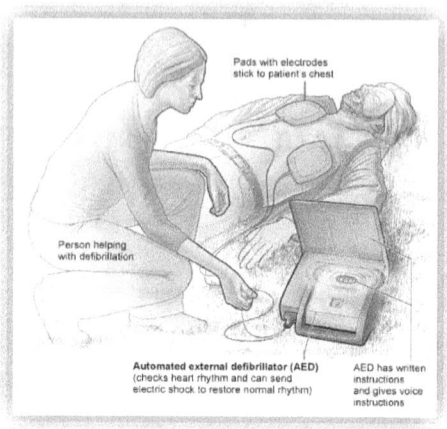

Pads with electrodes stick to patient's chest

Person helping with defibrillation

Automated external defibrillator (AED) (checks heart rhythm and can send electric shock to restore normal rhythm)

AED has written instructions and gives voice instructions

Figure 31: The typical setup using an automated external defibrillator (AED). IMAGE/ NIH

Step 6: Follow the AED's prompts to analyze the rhythm again after 5 cycles of CPR (about 2 minutes).

Step 7: Continue to monitor breathing if the victim recovers.

Special considerations:

➲ Do not use cellphone or two-way radio within 6 feet of an AED.

➲ Place the pads inches away if from an implanted defibrillator.

➲ AEDs require regular maintenance and replacement of batteries.

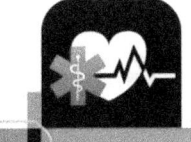

13.5 Ventilations

If a patient's breathing is not adequate or absent, you need to begin breathing for her immediately. You can assist breathing through mouth-to-mouth ventilation, hand-operated bag valve mask, or computerized ventilation machine.

Mouth-to-Mouth Ventilation

Mouth-to-mouth ventilation is the most basic and effective way of providing ventilation, where a rescuer presses their mouth against that of the victim and blows air (16% oxygen) into the person's lungs.

It generally entails providing air for a person who is not breathing or is not making sufficient respiratory effort on their own.

Many people are reluctant to perform mouth-to-mouth ventilation, often for fear of contracting deceases.

However, a number of pocket-size face shields and barrier devices are available which avoid mouth-to-mouth contact during ventilation. Polythene may also be modified with a small hole for blowing in air.

In hospitals and ambulances, medics use equipment like bag-valve-mask, supplemental oxygen or ventilator.

Bag Valve Mask

Bag-valve-mask (BVM) units are effective in providing ventilations to non-breathing victims.

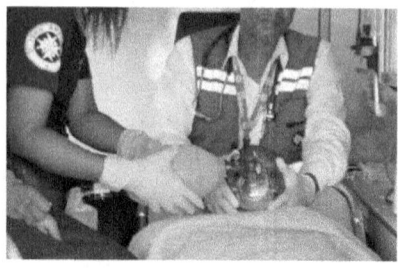

With the BVM, the casualty receives air from the atmosphere (21%), rather than from exhalation from the rescuer (16%).

BVM units have three main components:
- ⮑ Self-inflating bag holds oxygen that is delivered to the casualty when bag is squeezed.
- ⮑ One-way valve allows oxygen to flow to the victim, but prevents exhaled air from victim returning back to the bag.
- ⮑ Mask is connected to the bag and valve.

Using bag-valve-mask:

Step 1: Assemble the BVM, with correct mask size to cover the victim's mouth and nose.

Step 2: Open the airway and seal the mask to the victim's face.

Step 3: Squeeze the bag to provide ventilation. In adults, 1 ventilation in 5-6 seconds, and 1 ventilation in 3-5 seconds in infants.

Step 4: Recheck pulse and other signs of life about every 2 minutes. Call for an AED and begin CPR if there is no signs of blood circulation or breathing.

Ventilation Machine

A ventilator, is a machine that supports breathing by moving air into and out of the lungs.

Patients are placed on ventilators when they cannot breathe on their own. This may be to make sure the person is getting enough oxygen and is getting rid of carbon dioxide.

Most of the time, a ventilator is needed only for a short time. But in some cases, it is needed for months and at times years.

When a ventilator is used for more than a few days, the person may receive nutrition through tubes put in vein or stomach.

In its simplest form, the machine is attached to a computer with knobs and buttons. It also has tubes that connect to the person through a breathing tube.

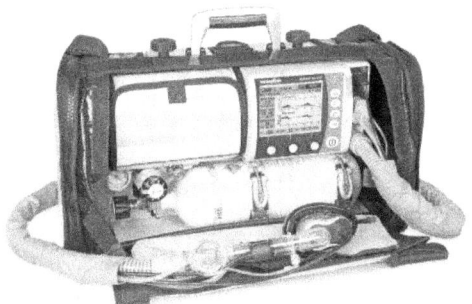

Usually, the breathing tube is put into the windpipe through the nose or mouth. It can also be placed in an opening through the neck into the windpipe (trachea). The patient-end of the circuit may be either non-invasive using masks or invasive using intubation.

Ventilators has alarms that alert when something needs to be adjusted.

Because the failure of a mechanical ventilation system may result in death, precautions must be taken to ensure that mechanical ventilation systems are highly reliable. This includes their power-supply provision.

Supplemental Oxygen

Supplemental oxygen is used along other life support techniques such as CPR. Victims of heart attack, stroke, seizures, or serious injury can also use supplemental oxygen.

Equipment involved in giving supplemental oxygen includes:
- ➲ Pressurized cylinder containing oxygen.
- ➲ Gauge showing the pressure remaining within the cylinder.
- ➲ Flowmeter, used to adjust the rate of oxygen delivery.

The following steps describe how to set up and give oxygen:

Step 1: Assemble the equipment: cylinder, flowmeter, tubing and delivery device ready.

Step 2: Remove any protective seal, while pointing the cylinder away, and open main valve for one second.

Step 3: Attach regulator to oxygen cylinder.

Step 4: Open the main cylinder valve and check the pressure regulator.

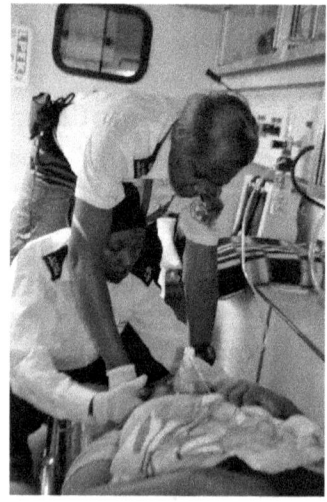

Step 5: Attach the tubing to the flowmeter.

Step 6: Set the flowmeter at the correct oxygen flow rate: 1-6 lpm for cannula, 10 lpm for face mask, and 10-15 lpm for BVM or non-rebreather mask.

Step 7: Confirm if oxygen is flowing.

Step 8: Apply the oxygen delivery device to the victim.

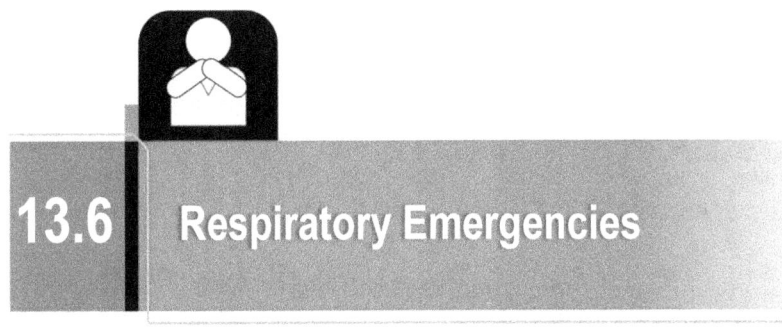

Breathing should be effortless and barely noticeable. If it is labored or noisy, too fast, or too slow, then it is not normal and should be treated promptly.

Where airway is totally obstructed, for instance in chocking cases, the victim has only 4-6 minutes, after which death can easily occur if proper first aid is not administered.

It is in this regard that people need to make first aid a must-have-skill, especially those taking care of small children who are quite vulnerable due weak anatomical structures.

These emergencies occur so fast that even the fastest ambulance may not reach the victim alive. The people around could be the only chance for lifesaving.

Some of the common respiratory emergencies have been highlighted below, including chocking, drowning and sudden instant deaths.

Obstructed Airway (Choking)

Chocking is one of the respiratory emergencies that occurs when airway is blocked by an object or dipping of tongue.

It often results from trying to swallow large pieces of food, eating too quickly, or eating while engaged in other activities.

Infants are more prone to chocking than adults due to weak body formation.

Chocking Care for Responsive Adult

The basic steps below highlight how to help a chocking adult:

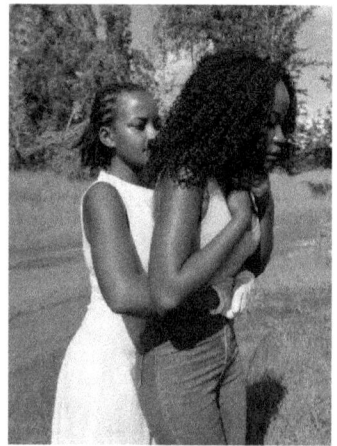

Step 1: Encourage coughing to clear obstructing object.

Step 2: Support the chest with one hand and give up to 5 back blows with the other.

Step 3: If the object does not come off, stand behind the casualty with one leg position between the victims legs.

Step 4: Make a fist with one hand and support with the other hand to thrust inwards and upwards on the abdomen just above the navel. Do this 5 times. For pregnant and obese victims, give chest compressions in the middle of the breastbone.

Step 5: Repeat 3 cycles of back blows and stomach thrust then call for an ambulance or rush casualty to hospital while continuing with chocking care.

In non-breathing and chocking victim, the chest compressions during CPR also helps to pressure out objects blocking the airway, in addition to resuscitating the heart.

If you are choking when alone, give yourself abdominal thrust using hands or leaning over and pushing your abdomen over the edge of a furniture to expel the object obstructing airway.

Chocking Care for Responsive Infant

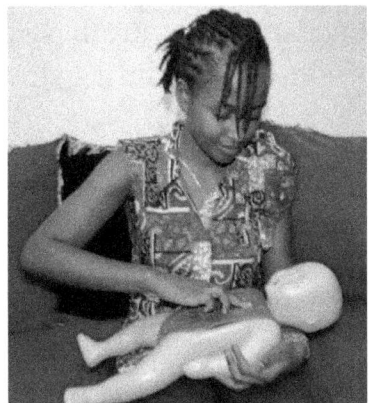

Step 1: Support infant's head with one hand and hold torso on your forearm or thigh.

Step 2: Check and remove any visible object using your small finger, but do not sweep blindly inside if you cannot see an object.

Step 3: Give up to 5 back blows with heels of your hand.

Step 4: If object does not come out of the mouth, give up to 5 chest thrusts using two fingers.

Step 5: Repeat 3 cycles of back blows and chest thrust then call for an ambulance or rush casualty to hospital while continuing with chocking care.

Prevent Chocking in Children and Infants

Children, especially infants below one year, are like vacuum cleaners, swallowing anything their hands bump on. Therefore take the following precautions:

- Do not leave toys that break off or small objects like buttons, coins and bids within reach of students.

- Have children sit at a table, rather than move around, while eating.

- Cut up foods a child may chock on, like hot dog, into small pieces.

- Supervise young children while eating, and be prepared with first aid skills to care for a child who chokes.

Sudden Infant Deaths (SIDs)

Sudden infant death syndrome (SIDS) is the unexplained death, usually during sleep, of a seemingly healthy baby less than a year old.

SIDS is sometimes known as crib death because the infants often die in their cribs.

To avoid sudden infant death syndrome:

- Place infants on their backs to sleep. Lying on the stomach may suffocate the nose and mouth with soft bedding.
- Remove toys and other soft objects from the baby's crib and never cover an infant's head during sleep to avoid suffocation.
- If blanket must be used, tuck it under edges of mattress below the chest level to reduce likelihood of infants pulling it over their face.
- When a woman smokes during pregnancy, the infant is three times more likely to have sudden infant death.
- Maintain a normal temperature in the infant's room, but do not overheat the infant.

Drowning

Drowning is another common respiratory emergency as nearly every river in Kenya has at one time or another been an agent of death through drowning.

Water related deaths also occur in flood water, swimming pools, bore holes, and even buckets, in the case of babies.

Breathing is impaired during drowning, as water close the airway and get into the lungs, preventing oxygen absorption.

Water Rescue

When you recognize a drowning victim, quick action is needed to rescue them.

The safest and most effective rescue technique is to reach the victim with some object, such as pole, that the victim can grasp while you pull them to safety.

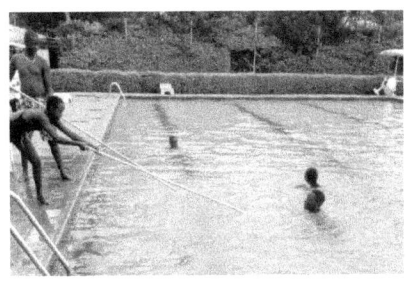

The second most effective technique is to throw a floating object, with a rope attached for pulling the victim to safety.

You should not go into water to rescue a drowning victim, unless you are trained and equipped. Most victims cling to anything tightly, and may hold your body, preventing swimming.

Caring for a Drowning Victim

Follow the following steps to care for a drowning victim once they are removed from water:

Step 1: Lie the casualty down, with their head slightly lower that the trunk of the body, to allow water to drain off by gravity. DO NOT compress stomach to remove water from casualty's body cavity.

Step 2: Open the airway and check for breathing.

Step 3: If resuscitation is necessary, give 5 initial rescue breaths. If the casualty is still not breathing, begin CPR as trained.

Step 4: If the casualty is breathing, place them on recovery position.

Step 5: Take off wet clothing and cover with blanket or warm clothing.

Step 6: If the victim becomes conscious, you can give warm (not hot) drinks, but not stimulants (alcohol or caffeine).

Step 7: All casualties of drowning must be taken for checkup in hospital to prevent secondary drowning.

Secondary drowning occurs when fluid that is breathed in irritates the lungs, and makes the airway swell and get narrower. This may occur several hours after the initial incident.

Aqua Safety

Water safety is important at any age to prevent drowning, but is especially crucial if you have babies or toddlers in your home or near water pools.

More than 90 percent of swimming pool drowning occur with an adult supervising, but distracted by other activities like talking on phone or reading.

Drowning can happen at home in filled bathtubs, swimming pools, and even buckets of water.

To reduce the risk of drowning, water safety is important at any age, but is especially crucial if you have babies or toddlers in your home.

The following are some of the aqua safety precautions:

- Avoid distractions, such as talking on mobile phone, while supervising children in a swimming pool.

- Do not drink near water. Alcohol impairs balance, and coordination which might lead to drowning.

- Swim with a buddy always. You may get help when drowning.

- Never leave a baby unattended in the bath. If you must answer the telephone or door, wrap your baby in a towel and bring him or her with you.

- Never leave any container filled with any amount of water or other liquid unattended.

- Keep bathroom doors closed at all times. (or you may want to install a doorknob cover)

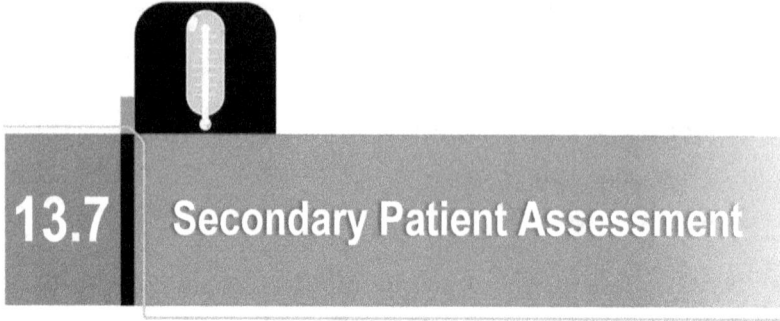

13.7 | Secondary Patient Assessment

After taking care of more urgent first aid procedures like opening airway, resuscitation and controlling heavy bleeding, secondary assessment is done to find out the mechanism of injury or nature of illness as well as medical history of the victim.

It is performed only for victims without life-threatening conditions. It provides additional information about the injury or illness.

The secondary assessment has two primary parts: Getting the victims history, and physical examination.

Getting the Victim's History

After the initial assessment, get the victims history to try to find out more about the victim's condition. Use SAMPLE technique to ensure you cover the victim's full history:

➲ **S**igns and symptoms you can observe.

➲ **A**llergies to food, medicines, or other substances.

➲ **M**edications being taken.

➲ **P**revious medical problems.

➲ **L**ast food and drinks taken.

➲ **E**vents leading to injury.

Talk to a responsive victim. If the victim is unresponsive, ask the family members or onlookers.

Physical Examination

Physical examination is done to assess the patient from top to toe to determine any other existing illness or injuries.

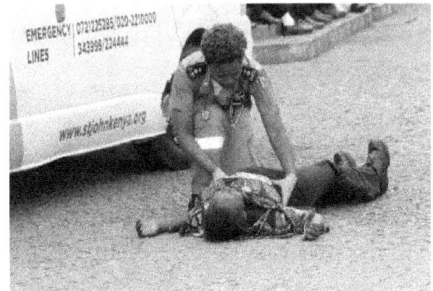

While conducting the assessment, allow a responsive victim to remain in their most comfortable position.

In adults, you may begin physical examination from the head, while in children, begin from extremities to slowly gain trust.

Talk to a child's parents or caretaker and involve them in physical examination to allow the child get used to you in nonthreatening manner.

While performing examination, look for pain, bleeding, deformities, abnormal movement, skin color, temperature and moisture.

Remove only necessary clothing while protecting the privacy of the casualty.

While checking the head for injuries, gently feel the skull, ears or nose for deformity, swelling, bleeding or pain. Check the pupil size, equality, and response to light.

To check for injuries at the torso, ask the casualty to take a deep breath and feel and look for uneasy, asymmetrical or pain on breathing.

Ask the casualty to bend knee and elbow and look for medical bracelets and necklace.

Assessing the Skin

Victim's skin provide important information about the flow of blood. For instance:

- Pale skin (whitish) occurs when blood vessels are severely narrowed.

- Cyanotic skin (blue-gray) suggests poor breathing or reduced blood flow to body tissues (perfusion).

- Jaundiced skin (yellow) may be seen in victims of liver or gallbladder problems.

- Hot skin may be caused by fever or heat exposure

- Localized warmth may be an indication of infection, inflammation, or burn.

- Wet or moist skin may indicate shock, heat-related illness, or diabetic emergency.

- Excessive dry skin may indicate dehydration.

- Capillary refill of 3-5 seconds on the nail bed may indicate poor blood flow or cold exposure.

To assess skin temperature, place back of your hand against the victims face, neck, or abdomen, and compare with your body temperature.

If available, thermometer may be used on the armpits, though rectal temperature gives the most accurate measure of temperature, however, it raises issues of sensitivity.

Assessing the Eyes

The pupils are normally equal in size, round and equally reactive to light. Briefly shine a light into the victim's eyes to assess the size, equality and reactivity of pupils.

Possible cause of:

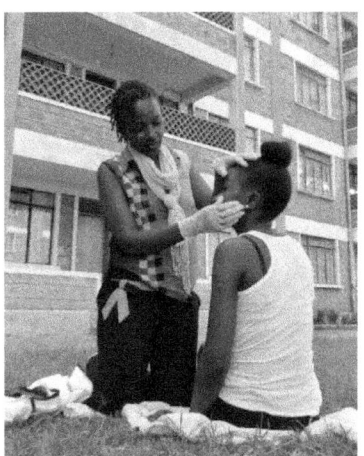

- Unequal pupils is stroke or head injury
- Non-reactive pupils is cardiac arrest or medication.
- Constricted pupils is narcotics, head injury or exposure to insecticides
- Dilated (very wide) pupils is trauma, fright, poisoning, or cocaine

Recovery Position

In unconscious victim who is breathing, and who is not suspected of having a spinal injury, should be put in recovery position.

The position helps to keep the airway open, allow fluids to drain from mouth, and prevent victim from inhaling stomach content if victim vomits.

To put casualty on recovery position, kneel on the casualty's left and place the arm near you at right angle then hold the arm furthest from you on his chick near you.

Pull the knee up of the leg furthest from you, and use it to roll the casualty towards you.

Laying the victim on their left side -rather than right side- reduces chances of vomiting due to anatomical differences inside the body.

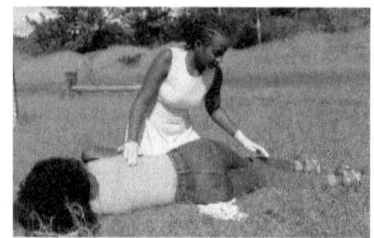

For infants and small children, hold the casualty face down over your arm with the head slightly lower than the body. Support the head and neck with your hand and keep the nose and mouth open.

13.8 Safe Lifting and Moving

A victim of an emergency is better off treated in the position they are found, and moved only when the following situations exist:

- There is danger, such as fire or flooding and you unable to protect the patient from the hazards.
- There are multiple patients and you need to reach the critically injured.
- Patient's location or position prevents providing lifesaving care.

The greatest danger of moving patients is the possibility of compounding spinal injuries, which can lead to fatality or paralysis. Always consider your safety first in all these situations.

Safe lifting means using your legs, not your back, and keeping your back as straight as possible when lifting a patient.

The following important guidelines can prevent injury when lifting, pushing or pulling:

- Consider the patient weight and need for additional help.
- Know your physical abilities and limitations.
- Before performing an emergency move, make sure the path is clear of obstructions.
- Mentally picture the patient's final position.

- When working with others, the person at the patients head directs the moves.
- Wear proper footwear, that maintain firm surface grip.
- Bend your knees, not your waist, and keep your back straight always.
- Use your legs, not your back to lift.
- Lift using smooth (not jerking) continuous motion.
- Walk slowly, looking where you are going.
- Push, rather than pull, whenever possible.
- When dragging a patient always pull along the length of the spine, and never pull the patient's head away from their neck or shoulder.

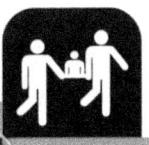

13.9 Emergency Moves

In the rare event that you need to provide an emergency move, realize that you will risk getting injured, as well as compound the patient's injury.

Some emergency moves include:

- ○ *Clothes drag*: Pulling the victim from the shoulder of their shirt.
- ○ *Blanket drag*: dragging the victim from the side under the head on a mattress or blanket.
- ○ *Ankle drag*: Slide your hand under the victim's armpit, and drug the casualty to safety.
- ○ *Firefighters drag*: used to move a patient from a smoke filled room. Tie the victim's wrist together, lift his arms over your neck, and raise your shoulders as you crawl forward so that the victim's head does not hit the ground.
- ○ *Firefighters carry*: Securing the victim in position on your shoulder.
- ○ *Cradle carry*: carrying small children on both your hands.
- ○ *Piggyback carry*: kneel for the victim to lean on your back with hands cross on your shoulders, then grab the knees as the victim holds tight across your chest.

- *Two person carry*: lock one arm to the other rescuer at the elbow to form a seat. Lock the other arm at the shoulder to hold the victim's back.
- *Human crutch*: act as a crutch by placing the victim's arm across your shoulder, and hold his wrist.
- *Two-person extremity lift*: one rescuer place arms under the victim's armpit and grab the victim's wrists. The second rescuer slips his hand behind the victim's knees, then both rescuers stand and move at the same time.
- *Stretcher* is the most common equipment used in stabilizing and moving victims. Stretchers work under the same basic principle with slight design and cosmetic variation. Different types include wheeled stretcher (common in ambulances), scoop stretcher, basket stretcher, canvas stretcher, stair chair, spine board (for spinal injuries), and vest-type (Kendrick) device.

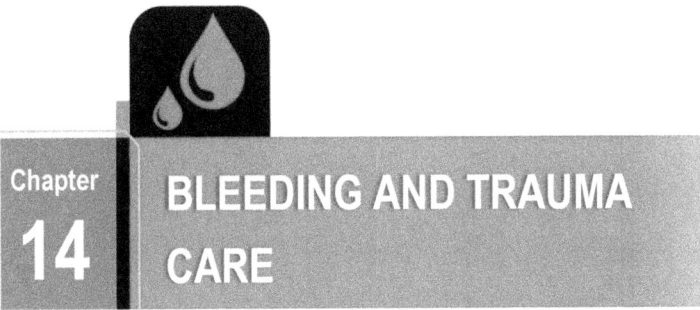

BLEEDING AND TRAUMA CARE

Penetrating trauma causes an open wound such as torn, cut, or punctured skin, while blunt force trauma causes a contusion (closed wound).

Generally, you cannot see closed wound. Therefore, it is important to consider the nature of injury when you assess the victim, and suspect internal bleeding with any injury involving a fall or moving locomotive.

A victim of internal bleeding may have cool clammy skin that is bluish, with possible confusion.

Deeper internal bleeding cannot be controlled by first aid. For that reason, take the casualty to hospital immediately.

For major wounds, control bleeding with your gloved hand and apply tight dressing without stopping circulation. DO NOT clean or apply antibiotic ointment.

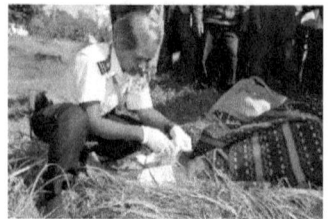

The pressure should be applied around, and not directly on the wound, to control blood loss in case of a skull fracture or objects spiked in the wounds.

If bleeding does not stop quickly, even after adding another bandage, then seek medical attention.

However, for open wounds and soft tissue injuries, the first aid care varies depending on their location in the body as highlighted below:

- For abrasions or shallow wounds, gently wash with soap on running water to remove dirt and cover with an adhesive plaster, sterile dressing or clean cloth.
- You can put cold pack on simple bruises to control bleeding, reduce swelling and pain.
- Always keep the injured part raised above heart level to reduce blood flow and swelling.
- Bleeding from a knocked out tooth may be controlled by pushing back the tooth into its socket or ask casualty to bite a gauze. Casualty should spit, not swallow blood.
- When bleeding from the ear, help the casualty in half sitting position, and hold a gauze against the ear and allow the fluid to drain on it.
- For nosebleeds, stop the blood loss by pinching the nose on the soft part for 10 minutes and bending with head forward to allow blood drain from nostrils.
- Apply airtight occlusive dressing, sealed on three sides, on sucking chest wound.

The following are key precautions to note during trauma care:

- Always protect yourself by putting on gloves or plastic bags or tell casualty to apply pressure with their own hand to prevent disease transmission.

- Sweating in a shock victim may not be a signal of extreme warmth, keep the victim warm with a blanket or coat.

- Do not remove heavy objects crushing a casualty after 15 minutes. This could cause instant death.

- Do not attempt to remove clothing stuck to a wound. Instead, cut around the clothing and leave it in place to be removed in hospital.

- Do not apply pressure on skull fracture or an object impaled in a wound. This may push in bones to pierce brain matter or release pressure holding bleeding at a major artery.

- Avoid breathing or blowing on the wound, since this may transmit pathogens.

- Refer all major wounds to hospital. A tetanus shot must be given within 72 hours of receiving a wound to be effective. Adults need a tetanus booster at least every 10 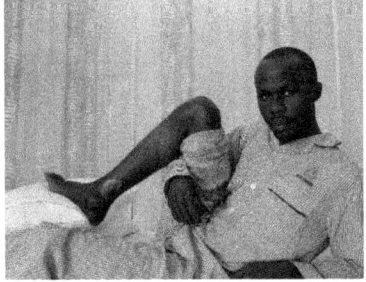 years, to reduce the impact of tetanus, which enters the skin through a wound, multiply, and produce a fatal toxins that acts on nervous system.

14.1 Shock (Severe Bleeding)

Severe bleeding is a life-threatening emergency, which if not controlled in time, can result in death or shock; a dangerous condition in which not enough oxygen-rich blood reaches vital organs like brain and heart.

Early signs of shock include restlessness, thirst, increased breathing and heart rate. The skin becomes pale and cool.

To treat shock:

- ⤷ have the victim lie on their back, raise the legs above heart level, loosen any tight clothing and cover the victim with a coat or blanket.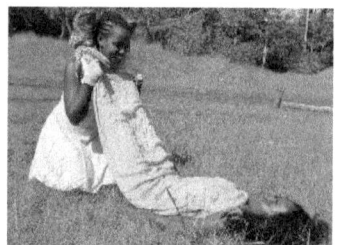

- ⤷ Sweating in a shock victim may not be a signal of extreme warmth, keep the victim warm with a blanket or coat.

- ⤷ Dot give a victim of shock anything to eat, drink or smoke, this may delay advanced medical procedures at the hospital.

14.2 Dressings and Bandages

Dressings

Dressings are put on the wound to help stop the bleeding, prevent infection, and protect the wound while it is healing.

There are many types of dressing, including gauze, adhesive strips (such as Elastoplast), eye pads, occlusive dressing and trauma dressing.

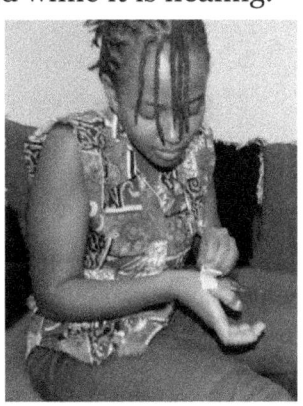

You can improvise a dressing by using clean non-fluffy cloth, or even sanitary pads.

Guidelines for using dressings:

Step 1: Wash hands and wear gloves.

Step 2: Open a sterile dressing larger than the wound without touching the part that will be in contact with wound.

Step 3: Carefully lay the dressing on the wound, without sliding it from side to side, to cover the whole wound.

Step 4: If blood seeps through, do not remove the dressing but add more dressings on top and apply a bandage to hold the dressing in place.

Step 5: Whenever you apply a bandage, check the victims skin color and sensation, to be sure that it is not too tight to cut off blood circulation.

Step 6: Keep fingers and toes open to check for circulation, discoloration or swelling when applying bandages.

Step 7: Avoid bending a joint once it has been bandaged because movement may loosen dressing or cut off circulation.

Bandages

Bandages are used for covering dressing and maintaining pressure to control bleeding.

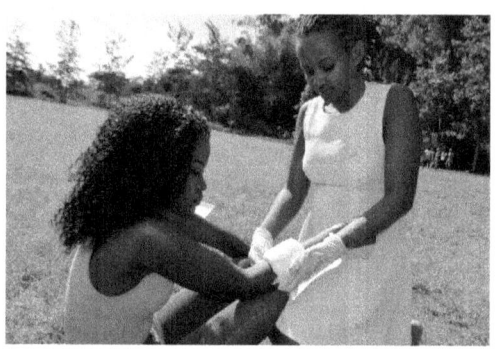

Bandages are also used to support or immobilize injury to bones, joints, or muscles and to reduce swelling.

Common types of bandages include: adhesive tapes, elastic bandage, roller bandage, and triangular bandage.

Any cloth can be improvised for use as a bandage.

Follow this guidelines for bandaging:

- Apply the bandage firmly, but not so tightly that it cuts off the blood flow.

- Do not cover the fingers or toes, unless they are injured. Keep them exposed to check blood flow.

- Keep checking the tightness as swelling continues after many injuries.

- An elastic bandage is used to support a joint and prevent swelling.

- Wrap a bandage from the bottom of the limb upward to avoid cutting off circulation of blood.

- Avoid bending a joint, once it has been bandaged because movements may loosen the dressing or cut off circulation of blood.

14.3 | Injury Prevention

W ounds may occur anywhere in the body as a result of any kind of trauma. Following are the general guidelines for injury prevention:

- ⮕ Always follow workplace safety guidelines when using machines and power tools to prevent injuries.

- ⮕ Wearing appropriate protective equipment like helmets, eye shields, gloves, and boots at work to prevent injuries.

- ⮕ Wear mouth guard in any activity that can result to a blow to the face or mouth, such as boxing or rugby.

- ⮕ Wear pelvic guard when participating in contact sports to prevent genital injury.

- ⮕ Women should wear a sports bra during exercises to prevent stretching, tearing of ligaments and supportive breast tissues.

14.4 Special Wounds

In addition to general guidelines for wounds, certain types of wounds require special first aid considerations. These include impaled object, amputations, genital injury, eviscerations, penetrating chest wounds and others.

Impaled object on wound

Removing an object from a wound could cause more bleeding and injury, as the object often seals the wound or damaged blood vessels.

Guidelines for care:

Step 1:   Control bleeding from impaled object wounds by applying direct pressure at the sides of the object.

Step 2:   Use bulky dressings or folded clothes to stabilize an impaled object and keep it from moving.

Step 3:   Take casualty to hospital.

Avulsions and Amputations

Avulsion is a part of skin torn partially from the body, like a flap. Move the tissue back to its normal position, unless it's contaminated; control bleeding; and provide wound care.

In an amputation, control the bleeding and care for victim's wound first, then recover and care for the amputated part.

Wrap amputated part in a sterile dressing or clean cloth, seal it in a watertight bag, and place in iced water.

Genital care

To control bleeding at the genitals, apply direct pressure using sanitary pads or sterile dressing, then secure with a diaper or triangular bandage.

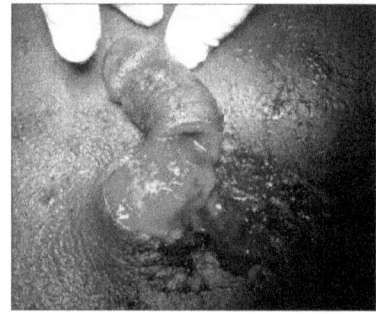

For blunt trauma on the testicles, a cold pack may help reduce pain. You may provide support with a towel between the legs, like a diaper.

For vaginal bleeding, have the woman press a sanitary pad or folded towel to control bleeding in the area.

In case of sexual abuse, preserve the evidence by asking victim not to urinate, bathe, or wash any area involved in the rape or assault.

Provide privacy for a victim when giving first aid for a wound in the genital area.

As a first aider, you must not visually inspect the vaginal area unless major bleeding is present, or you anticipate that childbirth is about to occur.

Penetrating chest wounds

This type of injury result from penetrating gunshot wounds, stabbings, blast injuries or impaled objects.

Air will enter through chest wound, rather than through windpipe, if chest wound is more than two-thirds the diameter of victims windpipe.

You may hear a sucking or gurgling sound escaping from the chest wound as the patient breathes in, signifying a life-threatening injury.

Cover sucking chest wounds with an occlusive dressing, or airtight rectangular wrap, taped on the three sides to prevent air moving in, while the open end allow air to escape when casualty breathes out.

Eviscerations

When an organ, like intestines, sticks out through an open wound:

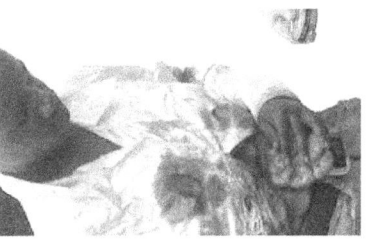

Step 1: Cover the organ with thick, moist dressing.

Step 2: Call for an ambulance immediately!

Step 3: Keep the patient in a position of comfort, usually with knees bent, if no spinal injury is suspected.

Step 4: Do not touch or try to place the exposed organ back into the body.

Neck injuries

Neck contains important airway structures, and swelling can cause airway obstruction.

A penetrating injury to the neck can result in severe bleeding, because the neck contains a major blood vessels.

To care for open neck wound:

Step 1:   Place a gloved hand over the wound to control bleeding, cover the wound with an airtight dressing taped on the three sides, and apply bulky dressings.

Step 2:   While applying pressure, make sure not to press on the windpipe or carotid arteries supplying blood to the head and brain.

Step 3:   Apply a pressure bandage across the injured part of the neck and under the opposite armpit. Never apply a bandage round the neck, it may cause strangulation.

Eye injuries

If foreign body or chemical is in the eye:

Step 1:   Gently flush it out with running warm water for at least 20 minutes from the nose-side of the affected eye.

Step 2:   If the object does not wash out of the eye, lift it with a clean, moist cloth, or transport casualty to hospital.

Step 3:   If foreign body is protruding from the eye, stabilize it then cover with a cup secured with a tape, and arrange for transport to nearest hospital.

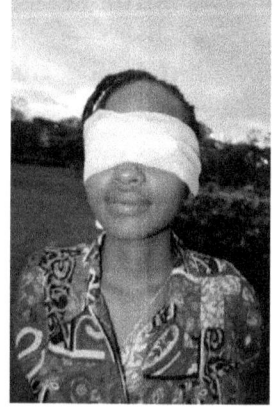

Step 4:   Because both eyes move together, you may cover the uninjured eye with a dressing as well.

Step 5: Irrigate the injured eye with plenty of water, for at least 20 minutes, in case of chemical burns. Alkali burns like lime and cement are more dangerous than acid burns like battery acid.

Step 6: Put a cold pack, but do not put pressure, over the eye if it is bleeding or leaking fluid for up to 15 minutes to reduce pain and swelling.

Mouth injuries

The tongue may fall back, blocking the airway, because of a lower jaw fracture, as it is attached to it.

Have a casualty bite a folded gauze into a removed tooth socket for 30 minutes to control bleeding. For a penetrating lip wound, roll a dressing between lip and gum and hold a second dressing outside the lip.

When bleeding stops, tell the victim not to drink anything warm for several hours. Do not let a victim swallow blood, which may cause vomiting.

Dentures or teeth should be placed in milk, and taken to a dentist with the casualty if they are found in the mouth.

Ear injuries

Suspect skull fracture if you see blood or clear fluid draining out of a victims ears. To care for ear injuries:

- Place a sterile dressing or clean cloth loosely over the ear to absorb blood drainage from the ear and bandage it in place.

- If the ear is completely cut off, cover it in a sterile dressing, seal in a watertight bag, and store in iced water to hospital.

Nosebleeds

To stop nosebleeds, have the casualty sit with head tilted forward, then pinch the fleshy part of the nostrils for 10 minutes, release and pinch again if bleeding continues.

Rush casualty to hospital if nose bleeding continues for more than 30 minutes.

Casualty should avoid breathing through the nose, sniffing or speaking during nose bleeding as this may disturb any clots.

Advice casualty to rest for few hours once nose bleeding has stopped then gently clean around the area with clean water.

Head and face wounds

Any significant injury to the head may signify spinal injury, therefore do not move casualty's head when giving first aid.

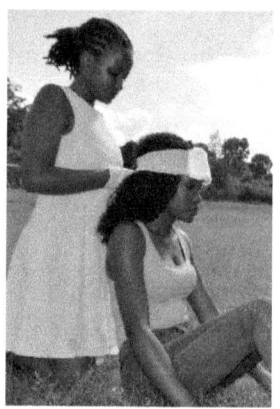

In case of scalp wound without suspected skull fracture, replace any skin flaps and apply direct pressure with gloved hand or sterile dressing, then bandage round the head.

14.5 Head and Spinal Injuries

Head and spinal injuries may cause death or permanent disability if not handled appropriately.

Motor vehicle crashes is the leading cause of spinal injuries. Other causes include sports activities, fall from tall structures and assault.

Unequal pupils, clear fluid from the ears and altered mental status are sure signs of brain injury. Other signs include headache, bleeding and deformities.

Inability to move any part of the body is a sure sign of spinal injury. Other indications include tingling, numbness or lack of feeling on the feet and hands.

When assessing head and spinal injury, check head and neck for deformity, swelling or pain, touch fingers and if sensation is normal, ask victim to push toes against your hand, make a fist and squeeze your hands.

Unless it is necessary to avoid eminent danger, do not move a victim with suspected spinal injuries.

In case of skull fracture, control bleeding by applying pressure round the edges, not on the wound, using gloved fingers or ring dressing.

All victims of spinal injuries should be secured on a flat backboard and transported in an ambulance. Manually stabilize the neck and head as you wait for an ambulance.

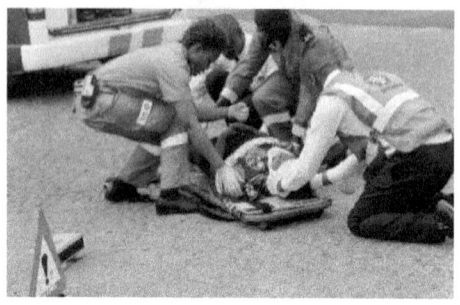

Inline stabilization means preventing movement of the head by supporting it in line with the body. Hold the victims head with both hands to prevent movement of the neck and spine, monitor breathing, and if needed, use soft objects like mattress block, to maintain support.

Use log-roll technique with at least three rescuers, to roll the victim and stabilize on a flat backboard. Rescuer at the victim's head directs others to roll the body as a unit.

All victims of head injury, however mild, should be diagnosed thoroughly in hospital, because it is generally difficult to determine seriousness of head injury from mere physical observation. It might have cumulative fatal effect.

Do not raise legs, or put a victim of spinal injury into recovery position.

14.6 Spinal Stabilization Techniques

Y ou may be required to assist a patient with spinal injuries. Equipment used for stabilization include: cervical collar, spine board, straps, tapes, and bandages.

If cervical collars are not available, the victims head can be stabilized by using a back board, rolled towels or blanket.

Three person log roll

This technique is used to roll a victim while keeping the head and neck in line with the rest of the body.

It is important to explain all movements to the victim, since he will have limited sight once immobilized on the board.

Step 1: Put on appropriate protective equipment, including gloves.

Step 2: First rescuer, giving all directions, holds the head in line with the rest of the victim's body.

Step 3: Second rescuer sizes and lace a rigid cervical collar.

Step 4: The second and third rescuer position the spine board at one side of the victim, then moves to the other side.

Step 5: The second rescuer places one hand on the victims shoulder and the other arm on the upper thigh.

Step 6: Third rescuer places one hand on the victim's hip and the other hand on the lower leg.

Step 7: When everyone is ready, the first rescuer, holding the head gives order to roll the victim at the count of 1...2....and..3!

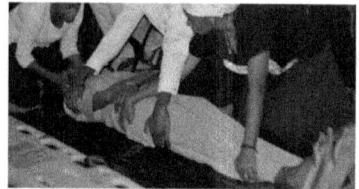

Step 8: While keeping the victim's head, shoulder, and pelvis in line, the second and third rescuers roll the victim to their side, while the first rescuer maintain inline stabilization of the head and neck.

Step 9: Using one hand from the lower leg, the third rescuer quickly assess the victim's back, and position the spine board under the victim.

Step 10: The first rescuer then gives command to roll back the victim onto the spine board.

Step 11: Manual stabilization of the head and neck is continued until the victim is fully immobilized on the spine board.

Spinal stabilization of a sitting victim

There are several types of short backboard used to immobilize a sitting victim, mostly in vehicle accidents.

Step 1: Put on appropriate personal protective equipment.

Step 2: First rescuer manually stabilizes the head in line with the other parts of the victim's body.

Step 3: Second rescuer assesses the victim's pulse, movement and sensation in all the extremities.

Step 4: After assessing the front and back of neck, a cervical collar is applied on the victim.

Step 5: Second rescuer places the vest-type device behind the victim, and fasten all the straps without interfering with the breathing.

Step 6: The victim is rotated so that his back faces the exit, and lowered on a long back board.

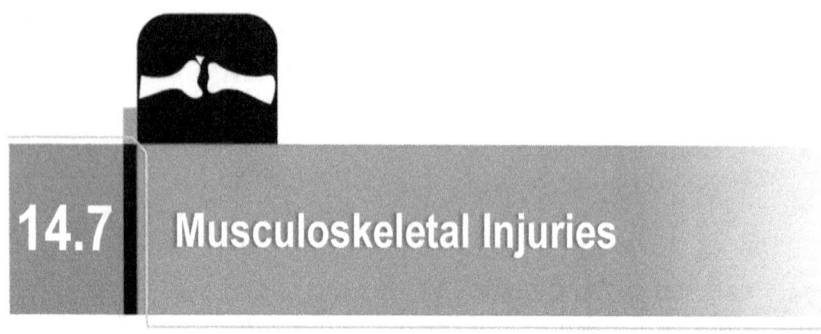

14.7 Musculoskeletal Injuries

The injuries result from forces acting on the bones, muscles and joints resulting in fractures, dislocations, strains, cramps, contusion, bone and muscle injuries.

Assessing Musculoskeletal Injury

Check for pain, swelling and bleeding when assessing an injured leg or arm. Other signs to look for include deformity, discoloration, sensation, and temperature.

Remove gently or cut off a victim's clothing to examine injuries and provide appropriate first aid care.

Lack of sensation and pain in an obviously injured area is a clear indication of nerves damage.

Swelling occurs in most injuries because of bleeding, but the amount of swelling is not a clear indication of severity.

Discoloration, usually blue-black, along with cool skin is an indication of lack of blood flow in the injured area.

General First Aid for Musculoskeletal Injuries

General first aid for most bone, joint and muscle injuries involves four steps acronym as PRICE - Protect injured part with a splint, Rest, Ice, Compress with elastic bandage, and Elevate above heart level.

There are several other acronyms like RICE, PIE, and PIES (pressure, ice, elevate, splint), but what matters of course is remembering the first aid technique behind the acronym.

Resting reduce bleeding and promote recovery of injured leg or arm.

Icing, especially with cold pack, numbs the nerves, reduce pain, and relieve muscle spasm. Ordinary ice wrapped in a cloth can also be used.

Cold works best if applied in the first 10 minutes after injury. Thereafter apply for 20 minutes after every hour.

Compression of a musculoskeletal injury, especially with an elastic bandage, provides comfort and prevents swelling.

Though commonly used, scientific findings have not confirmed any benefit or harm of compression in reducing swelling and bleeding.

Heat is also beneficial in treating sprains and strains, but should only be used after three days, after the initial swelling is diminished by cold treatment.

People sometimes get confused about applying cold, because they also know heat is used to treat musculoskeletal injuries.

After the third day, heat would encourage circulation and promote body's healing process.

The compression bandage should be firm, but not impede blood circulation. Loosen the bandage in case of discoloration or cool temperature.

Elevation of an injured arm or leg above the pumping heart uses gravity to slow blood flow, and reduce swelling and bleeding.

Elevation sling using a triangular bandage is often used on injured arm.

It's important to practice application of splints.

Muscle crumps, usually common on the thighs and calf is treated by stretching out the muscle if possible, and messaging the muscle after active cramping stops.

Fractures and Dislocation

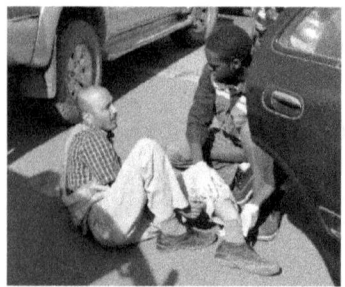

A fracture is a break or crack in the bone, while dislocation occurs when 2 bones are out of place at the joint that connects them. These may also cause injury to nerves and blood vessels.

Guidelines for first aid care:

- If the broken bone is the result of major trauma or injury, call local ambulance services.

- DO NOT encourage the casualty to move the injured part in order to identify a fracture.

- Examine the injured area for swelling or deformities, lacerations and puncture wounds. Gently feel along the length of the bone for tenderness, swelling and deformities.

- If you are not sure whether a bone is fractured, treat the injury as if it is.

- Stop any bleeding by applying pressure to the wound without causing further trauma. Dress wounds before applying a splint or sling.

- ⮑ Use a splint and immobilize the joints, above and below any fracture.

- ⮑ Apply ice packs to help limit swelling and relieve pain.

- ⮑ Treat for shock if necessary.

- ⮑ Check for a pulse and sensation below the fracture area.

Muscle Cramp

Muscle cramps are a common, especially in the legs and feet.

It is sometimes caused by dehydration (loss of water) and low levels of potassium, in hot weather, when your body loses water, salt, and minerals through sweating.

Drinking plenty of water and eating foods rich in potassium, such as bananas, may help to ward off cramps.

You can also get a cramp while exercising, particularly if you do too much. But cramps can even occur when you're sleeping.

Older people are more susceptible to muscle cramps due to less active life, and the natural muscle loss that begins in mid-40s.

Most muscle cramps don't last very long, though some can go on for 15 minutes or longer.

If you do get muscle cramps, the following simple tips can ease the pain and loosen the cramp:

Step 1: Stretch while gently massaging the cramped muscle.

Step 2: If the cramp is in your calf muscle, bring your foot up toward your shin.

Step 3: If the cramp is in the front of your thigh, bend your knee and pull your foot toward your buttocks.

Step 4: Hold the stretch until the cramp subsides.

Step 5: Drink water or a sports drink.

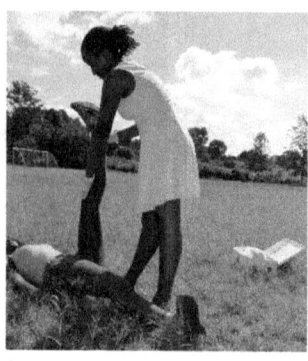

Step 6: For tight, rigid muscles, apply deep heat.

Step 7: For muscles that are tender or sore, which may be inflamed, applying ice may help.

Hamstring Injury

Hamstring injury is common in sports. It occurs when hamstring muscles are torn if forcibly stretched beyond limits.

The immediate treatment of a Hamstring muscle injury consists of the RICE protocol - Rest, Ice, Compression and Elevation. (never apply ice directly to the skin)

Resting may be the common sense approach, but it is one that is often ignored by competitive athletes. This is unwise, since it can turn the Hamstring strain from bad to worse.

Regardless of the severity of the injury, hamstring should be rested in an elevated position with an Ice Pack applied for 20 minutes every two hours. (never apply ice directly to the skin).

A Compression Bandage should be applied to limit bleeding and swelling in the tissues.

You may want to use over the counter anti-inflammatory medication, such as diclofenac to reduce pain.

There has been some controversy that these medications stop pain, but also may stop a phase of chemical reactions that are important in long term healing.

Therefore, some doctors recommend their use starting 48 hours after the injury.

As a general rule, Hamstring strains should be rested from sporting activity for about 3 to 6 weeks.

In the case of a complete rupture, the Hamstring muscle will have to be repaired surgically and the rehabilitation afterwards will take about 3 months.

Prevention of Sports Injuries

Preventing sports injuries begin with correct use of sports equipment such as boots, chin guards, helmets, or pelvic guards, and following rules of the game.

- Warm up before sporting activities.

- Cool down following sporting activities.

- Stretch regularly to maintain muscle length.

- Replenish carbohydrates during sporting activity with glucose.

- Wear compression shorts or thigh support to retain muscle warmth.

- Avoid playing sports or exercising when tired or in pain.

- Maintain healthy diet, weight, and stretch exercises to reduce risk of sports injuries.

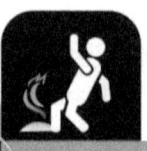

14.8 | Burn Care

A burn is damage to your body's tissues caused by heat, chemicals, electricity, sunlight, or radiation.

Although minor burns may damage only outer layer of the skin, more severe burns damage the middle or deeper layer containing nerves and blood vessels.

Burns extending deeper into the skin may expose it to infection, cause loss of body fluid and heat, or damage to organs under the skin.

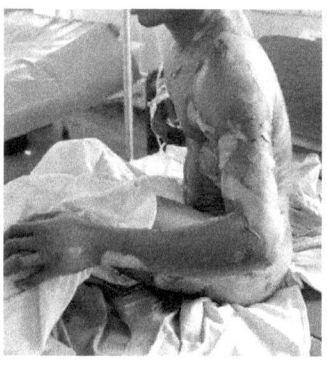

Burns to the middle skin layer is most painful due to nerves damage, however, there may be no pain on deeper layer burn as nerve endings are completely destroyed.

Steps for burn care:

Step 1: Skin keeps burning even if fire is out, so cool the burn areas with water immediately.

Step 2: Remove the victim's jewelry and constrictive clothing before swelling starts.

Step 3: Cover the burn with dry, loose, non-sticky dressing.

Precautions:

○ Do not apply ointment or other substances on all burns.

○ Do not break skin blisters; this could cause an infection.

○ Deep skin burns should not be cooled for more than 20 minutes, because of the risk of shock or cold emergencies like hypothermia.

Smoke Inhalation

Any victim in the vicinity of a fire could have swollen airway, damaged lungs, or carbon monoxide poisoning from inhaling smoke or other fumes.

Signs of smoke inhalation include coughing a sooty substance, difficulty breathing, and blackening around the mouth or nose.

Get the victim of smoke inhalation to fresh air or ventilate area by any means, and help them into position of comfort, often semi-reclining.

Chemical Burns

Protect your skin with gloves and irrigate the area with plenty of water for at least 20 minutes, remove jewelry from burn areas, and move victim to fresh air.

Cover the burn with loose, dry, non-sticky dressing.

Electrocution and Lightning Burns

Typical electrical injuries occur from faulty appliances, exposed power cords or when appliance comes into contact with water.

To prevent electrocution, always repair or replace damaged appliances, wiring, and avoid using electrical appliances anywhere they might come in contact with water.

Disconnect the source of electricity or pull casualty off using non-conductor material like dry wood or plastic. If you touch a person being electrocuted, you will get an electric shock too, and may also be injured.

The severity of an electrocution injury depends on the voltage. Shock from high voltage power lines can jump up to 18 meters and will nearly always kill.

In such high voltage electrocution, call Kenya Power to switch off power before starting to offer first aid.

Lightning or electricity may cause cardiac arrest. After power is switched off, give rescue breaths and chest compressions if there is no breathing, and treat other soft tissue injuries.

All lightning and electrical burns should be evaluated in hospital for damage to internal organs like lung or heart.

Look for entrance, usually dry and leathery, and exit wound, which is much larger and cover the burn with dry, loose, non-sticky dressing.

Ensure the following precautions:
- Keep children away from electric appliances.

- Check power cords regularly, making sure there are no exposed wires.

- Don't use electrical appliances in wet locations

- Don't overload power outlets with many appliances.

- Never forget - water and electricity don't mix!

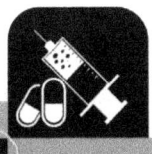

MEDICAL EMERGENCIES

Medical emergency refers to any health problem that could cause death or permanent injury if not treated quickly.

Common symptoms of such emergencies include shortness of breath, altered mental status, and loss of consciousness among others.

These emergencies usually require attention of a doctor, although some can be dealt with by the victim themselves or first responders.

Any medical emergency depend on the situation, the age of victim involved, and availability of the resources to help.

Some examples of medical emergencies are:

- Heart attack with symptoms like chest pain accompanied by sweating, nausea, vomiting, shortness of breath, radiating pain that moves to the arm or neck, dizziness, or feeling that your heart is beating irregularly or too fast.
- Stroke and altered mental status
- Asthma and allergies
- Fainting
- Seizures
- Diabetes
- Vomiting and diarrhoea
- Poisoning
- Bites and stings

A key component of providing care is to take the patient to hospital or call for ambulance services if available.

While calling for emergency help, note that the primary focus of any emergency or ambulance service is to treat the critically ill and injured first.

Patients seeking treatment of minor illnesses and injuries may be asked to wait for longer or be advised to use alternative transport such as taxis.

These minor illnesses and injuries are referred to as non-emergencies. They include:

- Head ache and fever that is relieved with over-the-counter medication
- Cold or flu symptoms and sore throat
- Earache and toothache
- Minor cuts, scrapes and abrasions,
- Muscle sprains, and
- Sunburn among others.

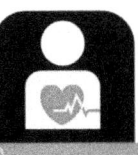

15.1 Heart Attack

Heart attack, also called acute myocardial infarction, involves sudden reduced flow of blood to heart muscles due to narrowing or tightening of blood vessels.

Over time, cholesterol and a fatty material called plaque can build up on the walls inside blood vessels that take blood to your heart. This makes it harder for blood to flow freely.

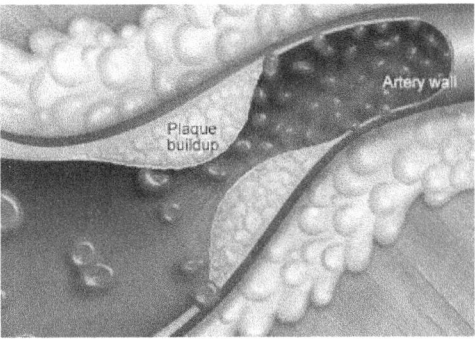

Most heart attacks happen when a piece of this plaque breaks off. A blood clot forms around the broken-off plaque, and it blocks the artery.

When blood can't get to your heart, your heart muscle doesn't get the oxygen it needs. Without oxygen, its cells can be damaged or die.

The key to recovery is to get your blood flow restored quickly. Get medical help right away if you think you're having symptoms of a heart attack.

Chest pains is still the common sign of heart attack, women are likely to have back pain and nausea.

Other signs include feeling of impending doom, sweating and greyish lips.

A victim may have no symptoms of heart attack at all before collapsing.

Act quickly during heart attack, because deaths occur within 1-2 hours after symptoms begin.

In case of heart attack, call an ambulance, place the casualty 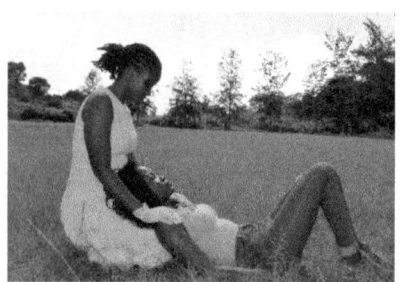 in a half sitting position with knees raised, reassure and allow victim to chew one aspirin if they do not have medication.

Nitroglycerin, a medication for heart attack, increases blood flow through the narrow blood vessels by dilating them, while aspirin makes blood thinner to pass through blood vessels.

Angina is also a heart disease with similar symptom and first aid treatment as heat attack. However the chest pain disappears within 10 minutes.

If breathing is absent, begin CPR immediately as you wait for an ambulance to arrive.

Preventing Heart Conditions

Heart attack can be caused by uncontrollable as well as controllable risk factors.

Uncontrollable risk factors include aging, male gender and hereditary factors.

Controllable risk factors are smoking, inadequate exercise, obesity, stress, high blood pressure and cholesterol levels.

To prevent the killer heart disease, reduce the risk factors by eating healthy diet, not smoking, getting exercise, maintaining normal weight, controlling stress and blood pressure.

Recent studies suggest that the best eating plans are based around vegetables, wholegrain and lean proteins. There are also a variety of healthy fats, like those from nuts, fish, avocados and olive oil.

Plant-based wholefoods tend to confer other benefits like reduced risk of diabetes and some types of cancer.

When it comes to quitting smoking tobacco, it's not easy to quit, as its nicotine content is highly addictive.

Almost all adults who smoke know that it is unhealthy, yet still have difficulty quitting.

But commitment to quitting, along realistic attitude and plan has led millions to successfully break the habit.

Although few children experience heart disease from very early age, they form habits like poor diet and passive leisure that often stay to haunt them for life.

Conduct regular checks for hypertension, often called silent killer, as the person can be completely unaware of having it, yet it is linked to high death rates caused by heart attack and stroke.

Hypertension shows no symptom and can be confirmed by systolic blood pressure test of above 120.

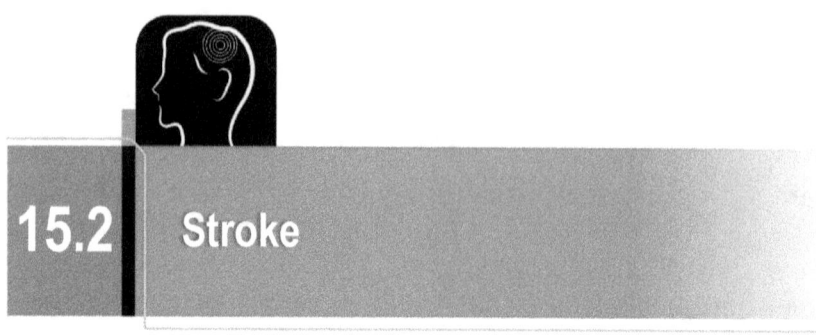

15.2 Stroke

Stroke is the interruption of blood flow to a part of brain, causing death of nerve cells. Transient Ischemic Attack is similar to stroke, only that symptoms disappears within a few minutes.

Stroke, like heart attack, may be caused by narrowing of blood vessels in the brain. Blood may clot in the artery or an artery may rapture in the brain.

Quick identification of the signs of stroke, and prompt treatment decrease the chance of permanent damage.

Typically, only one side of a stroke victim functions e.g. one side of face smiles, unequal lifting of hands, and slurred speech.

The most important thing to do for a stroke victim is to call for an ambulance or rush to hospital immediately, lay the victim down with back and shoulder slightly raised, loosen tight clothing, and reassure the casualty.

Drugs in hospital can minimize the effects of stroke, but only if administered very soon after the stroke.

15.3 Allergies and Asthma

Allergies

Anaphylaxis or massive allergic reaction is the inflammation of the airway, making breathing impossible.

It's the normal action of immune systems response to foreign substances (allergens) such as foods, drugs, bites and stings.

To prevent anaphylaxis, avoid substances that your body is allergic to and stay away from insect nesting areas, sweet smelling perfumes, waving away insects, and reptiles.

If stung by an insect, do not pull the stinger out using your fingers, instead scrap it off with something of similar size to credit card, to avoid injecting more venoms from venom sac.

Early signs of anaphylaxis include skin itching, rushes, feeling tickle on the throat, and altered mental status.

In case of massive allergic reaction, call for an ambulance, help the victim sit in position of easy breathing, help the victim use their epinephrine drug if they have.

Asthma

Asthma is the narrowing of the airway caused by allergens or irritants such as dust, fumes, extreme weather or emotional stress.

Asthma cannot be cured, but it can be managed.

Wheezing is the most common sign of asthma. Other symptoms include chest tightness, gasping for air, panting, bluish lips, and cool and moist skin.

In case of asthmatic attack, call for an ambulance, allow casualty to assume position of easiest breathing (often leaning forward), help the victim take his prescribed medication, reassure them to reduce anxiety and encourage patient to breathe deeply.

If available, assist the casualty to take their prescribed inhaler (bronchodilator) and transport to hospital. Never use another person's inhaler.

Bronchodilators or inhalers is a medication for asthma. It relaxes the muscles of the airway, allowing the airway to open wider and make breathing easier.

Guidelines for using inhaler:

Step 1:   Have the victim breath out fully,

Step 2:   Press the inhaler down while inhaling slowly and deeply, and

Step 3:   Hold breath for 10 seconds then exhale slowly.

Knowing the triggers that provoke asthma can help prevent asthmatic attacks. People with asthma should know what triggers the attack and such situations, and carry their medication with them.

Dust surfaces with dump cloth, avoid fluffy beddings, do not use strong air fresheners, and stay indoors when pollens are high.

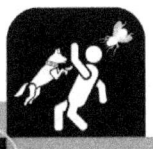

15.4 Bites and Stings

Bites and stings by animal, human and insects can result into a medical emergency such as allergy and bleeding.

Any animal that bites a person is assumed to have rabies, unless the animal can be killed and its brain examined for the virus.

First aid for bites by any organism focuses on controlling bleeding, wound care, and quick hospitalization.

If bitten by a dog, clean the wound with soap on running water for 5 minutes, apply pressure to control bleeding, cover wound with clean dressing, and visit hospital immediately.

Prevention of Dog Bites and Rabies

People keep dogs at home as pets, and for security. However, these canines wreck serious attack and cause fatal rabies, unless vaccination injections are given early in hospital.

The following precautions may prevent dog bites and rabies:

- Remain motionless, be still like a tree when approached by unfamiliar dog.

- Never approach, scream or run from strange unfamiliar dogs.

- Do not disturb a dog that is a sleep, eating or caring for puppies.

- Do not play aggressive games, such as wrestling, with a dog.

- Never allow children to play with dogs and pets, unless supervised by an adult.

- Never leave young children alone with a dog, as they have not learnt how to safely interact with pets.

- Consult with a veterinary officer to determine suitable breed of a dog based on your lifestyle and environment.

- Exclude dogs with history of aggression from households with children.

Snakebites

People living in areas where venomous snakes are common should take preventive steps and know what first aid to give in case bite occurs.

Treat all snake bites as potentially dangerous, unless you are very certain that a bite was from a non-venomous snake.

If bitten by a snake, have the victim lie down and stay calm, wash the bite with soap, wrap the extremity with an elastic bandage (not too tight), and remove any jewelry before swelling occurs.

Do not try to catch the snake, but note its appearance and describe to hospital doctor. You can take a picture of the snake if you have a camera, without endangering yourself.

Many traditional myths such as sucking the wound or tying the leg with a rope do not in fact improve the victim's condition.

To prevent snakebites:

- Stay away from underbrush areas, fallen trees and other areas where snakes may live.

- If you see a snake, reverse your direction and retrace footsteps, watching for other snakes.

- Beware of peak movement times. Most reptiles are active during warm months.

- Never handle a venomous reptile, even if it is dead.

- If untrained, never try to capture or harass reptiles.

- Use protective gears, such as gumboots and industrial gloves when slashing or clearing thickets.

Insect Bites

Insect bites may cause massive allergic reaction besides pain and swelling at the point of bite.

If a victim of insect bite has difficulty breathing, call for an ambulance, keep the bite area bellow the heart, wash the area with soap, and cool with an ice pack.

Bee and Wasp Stings

Insect stings are not poisonous but can cause life-threatening allergic reactions.

Scrap off stinger gently with a piece of plastic, wash area with soap, reduce pain and swelling with ice, and watch for any signs of allergy.

Do not scratch or use fingers to remove stinger as this may squeeze more venoms increasing swelling, itching and infection.

Over the counter antihistamine medication may help reduce discomfort.

A victim of insect sting in the mouth or on the lips may suck ice to reduce swelling.

Most people who are allergic to bites and stings carry EpiPen medicine. Help them to use the medication.

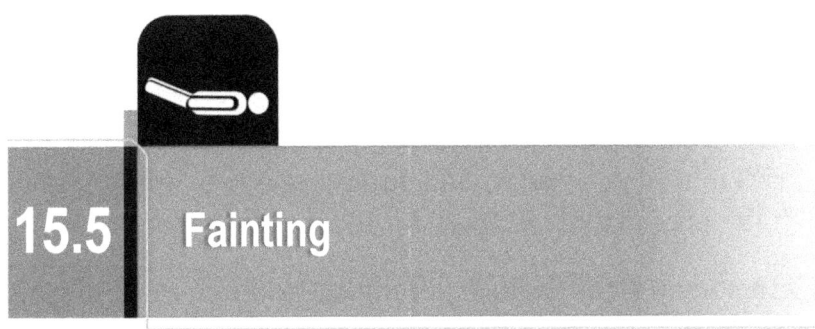

Fainting or syncope is a sudden, brief loss of consciousness and posture caused by decreased blood flow to the brain.

The brain relies on oxygen carried in the blood to function properly. Fainting can occur when the blood flow to the brain is reduced.

Your body usually corrects reduced blood flow to the brain quickly, but it can make you feel sweaty and dizzy. If it lasts long enough, you may faint.

Reduced blood flow to the brain is often caused by a temporary problem with the part of your nervous system that regulates the body's automatic functions, including heartbeat and blood pressure.

It can also occur in hot weather, prolonged activity, or lack of food.

If you feel you're about to faint, lie down, preferably in a position where your head is low and your legs are raised. This will encourage blood flow to your brain.

Most cases of fainting aren't a cause for concern and don't require treatment, but less common types of fainting can be medical emergencies.

But fainting may be a sign of serious problem requiring medication in a person with heart disease, pregnant women and elderlies.

Injuries may also occur when a fainting person falls, so try to catch the person and gently lower them to the floor.

Have a person sit or lie down if fainting is anticipated by signs like nausea, dizziness, blurring vision, and general weakness.

In case of fainting, lay the victim down, raise legs, loosen constricting clothing, check for possible injuries caused by falling, and reassure as they recover.

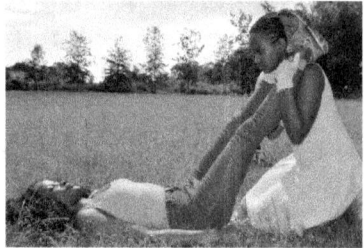

Call for an ambulance if the victim does not regain responsiveness or faints repeatedly.

Do not pour water on the victims face, it could be aspirated into the lungs.

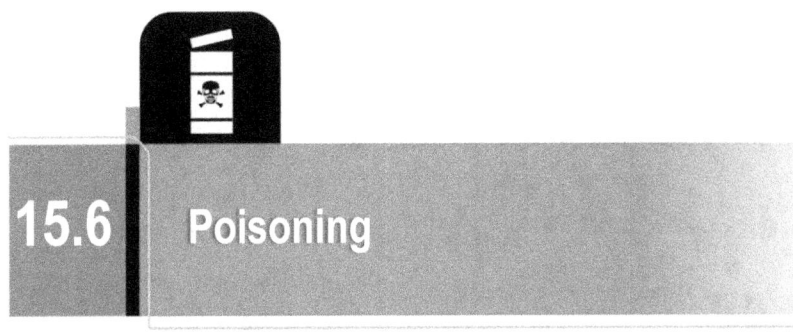

15.6 Poisoning

Most poisonings are accidental, occurring in the home to children under the age of six.

The potential for these accidental poisonings has been dramatically affected by changes in our society.

Such changes include increase towards single parent families and families in which both parents work outside of the home, leaving housemaids and children in charge of younger siblings.

Common poison exposures for children are swallowing of household products, suicide attempts in teens, and pain relievers in adults.

Carbon monoxide, mostly from using charcoal jikos in enclosed room, is especially very lethal because it's invisible, odorless, and tasteless.

A poison is any substance that can harm someone if used in the wrong way, by the wrong person or in the wrong amount.

It can enter the body through swallowing, injection, inhalation, absorption.

Anything taken in excess can also be poisonous, including food, and prescribed or over the counter medication.

Alcohol poisoning causes the most poisoning deaths in Kenya.

Consumption of illicit brews is so prevalent to an extent

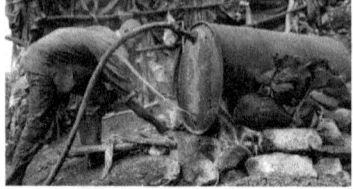

consumers literally live in the dens of the deadly concoctions, oblivious of its fatal consequences, including blindness.

Figure 32: Preparing illicit brew

The brews, said to be laced with body-preservation chemicals, notably formalin and ethanol, are highly intoxicating.

Cases of drink-spiking in pubs is also increasingly worrying, particularly male revelers who are the main targets.

General First Aid for Poisoning

The most common symptoms of poisoning include nausea, vomiting abdominal pain and diarrhea.

In most cases you'll not know the specific treatment for a poison. But the first steps in a poisoning emergency is to call for an ambulance, or seek alternative transportation to hospital.

Meanwhile, you can conduct the following first aid procedures:

- ➲ Eyes: Flood eye with clean water for at least 20 minutes. Do not force the eye to open.

- ➲ Skin: Remove contaminated clothing and flood skin with water for at least 20 minutes. Then wash gently with soap and water and rinse.

- ➲ Mouth: Do not give anything by mouth. This may delay surgical procedure.

- **Corrosive Chemicals:** Unless patient is unconscious or having convulsions, give sips of milk or water.

- **Swallowed Poison:** determine the poison, and rush the casualty to hospital immediately. Activated charcoal, which absorbs some kinds of poison, may be used only if advised by a Doctor.

- **Food Poisoning:** let the victim rest lying down, give lots of clear fluid, and seek immediate medical attention in hospital.

- **Inhaled Poison:** Whenever you smell a toxic gas or have other evidence of leaked toxic fumes, stay away from the scene. Move the casualty outdoors for fresh air, but do not risk your own health if scene is dangerous.

- **Unresponsive Victim:** place the victim in recovery position, and loosen tight clothing around neck or chest.

- **NEVER** make the victim vomit. It can be dangerous to induce vomiting.

Preventing poisoning

Most poisoning can be prevented by observing the following precautions:

- Store potential poisons out of reach of small children.

- Store all products in their original containers and return household chemicals to safe storage after use.

- Keep children out of places sprayed with pesticides, they can be absorbed through the skin.

- Do not take medicine in front of children. Young children often imitate adults.

- Know the plants in your home, some may be poisonous such as potato plant leaf.

- Store food and household chemicals separately. Mistaken identity could cause a serious harm.

- Read and follow cautions and instructions on household chemicals.

- Open windows when using chemicals.

- Never sniff containers to detect what is inside.

- Whenever you smell a toxic gas or have other evidence of leaked toxic fumes, stay away from the scene.

Preventing drink-spiking

To reduce the risk of drugging and secondary crime such as rape and kidnapping, the following precautions are recommended:

- Do not leave your beverage unattended in a social setting.

- When you go to party, go with a group of friends, watch out for each other, and leave together.

- Beware of your surroundings at all the times.

- Don't allow yourself to be isolated by someone you don't know.

- Think about the level of intimacy you want in a relationship, and clearly state your limits.

Preventing Food Poisoning

- Refrigerate foods promptly. Unrefrigerated food left for 2 hours is unsafe for eating.

- Cook food to appropriate temperature to kill harmful bacteria.

- Handle food properly. Always wash your hands before touching food and after visiting the washroom.

- Keep cold food cold and hot food hot.

- Refrigerate cooked perishables, prepared food and leftovers within two hours.

- Do not overfill refrigerator. Cool air must circulate to keep food safe.

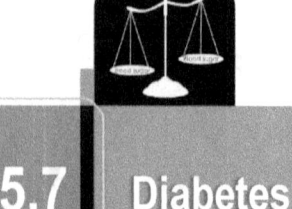

15.7   Diabetes

Diabetes is a condition in which the blood sugar levels are not regulated well by the body. The pancreas may not produce enough insulin, or the body may not use insulin well.

Normally, the pancreas (an organ behind the stomach) releases insulin to help your body store and use the sugar and fat from the food you eat.

In a person with diabetes, the pancreas produces very little or no insulin. the body may also not respond appropriately to insulin.

At present, there is no cure, and people with diabetes need to manage their disease to stay healthy.

Control

Even though diabetes is incurable it can be controlled with diet, exercise, weight control, and medication.

If not managed well, diabetes may cause heart disease, stroke, blindness, severe kidney disease and damage to nervous system.

For those with diabetes, careful control of their glucose levels, blood pressure, and cholesterol levels can help prevent fatal complications.

Low Blood Sugar (Hypoglycemia)

Symptoms of low blood sugar (hypoglycemia) include sweating, altered mental status, staggering, or slurring of words like a drunk or intoxicated person.

First aid for hypoglycemia involves raising the person's blood sugar level by giving solution of sugar, food or drink that is high in glucose.

Diabetics often carry glucose tablets in case of low blood sugar.

Always take a victim of diabetes to hospital if they become unresponsive or continue to have significant symptoms.

Do not give food or drinks in the mouth of unresponsive diabetic victim.

High Blood Sugar (Hyperglycemia)

Fruity smelling breath is a clear sign of high blood sugar level, known as hyperglycemia. Other signs include drowsiness, shortness of breath, and frequent urination.

Hyperglycemia generally requires medical treatment in hospital.

If you cannot judge whether a victim has low or high blood sugar level, give sugar and seek medical care if the victim does not improve in 15 minutes.

It can be frightening to be with someone ill, especially if you do not know first aid. Always remember to call for an ambulance or other alternative transport, and do not give anything to eat or drink.

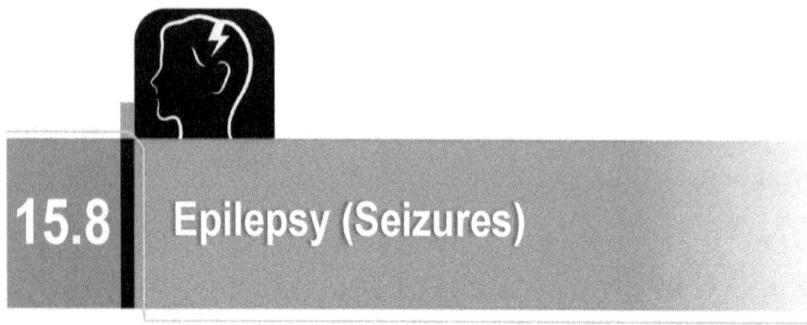

15.8 Epilepsy (Seizures)

E pilepsy is a disorder of the brain, in which a person experiences seizures as a result of disturbance of their brain's electrical activity.

However, many people still have a misconception that it is a result of curse, witchcraft, or that epileptic people are demon-possessed. Some also believe it's contagious, which is not true.

These negative beliefs at times stigmatize affected people and create barriers in their lifestyles.

At home, some people living with epilepsy are hidden by their parents to avoid 'shame,' denying them vital rights like going to school, which makes them develop low self-esteem.

To cope with such stigma, it's vital to have support from others who have the disorder and connect with the local Epilepsy Support group or a similar organization.

This is helpful in getting advices on proper diagnosis, medication, and dealing with the stigma.

Causes

Anyone can have a one-off seizure, but this doesn't always mean they have epilepsy. It's only diagnosed if someone has more than one seizure that is not caused by a known medical condition.

Possible causes of epilepsy include stroke, severe head injury, or brain infection like meningitis. But in over half of all people with epilepsy, the cause is not known.

Some may have a family history of epilepsy, suggesting that they may have inherited it.

Even so, it's not important to know the cause of seizure in order to manage a person who is having it.

Triggers

Triggers do not cause epilepsy itself, but they activates the shaking and jerking motions. Common triggers include:

- Not taking antiepileptic drugs as prescribed
- Not sleeping well
- Stress
- Alcohol and recreational drugs
- Flashing or flickering lights
- Monthly periods
- Missing meals
- Having an illness which causes a high temperature
- Low blood oxygen and sugar to the brain

Not all people with epilepsy have seizure triggers, and the things that trigger a person's seizures may not affect another.

After the trigger, some people experience an aura, which is a feeling or warning of an impending convulsion.

Prevention

A first time seizure cannot be prevented, but diagnosed disorder has prescribed antiepileptic drugs that suppress the seizure.

Nonetheless, seizures caused by head injuries can be prevented by wearing protective gears like helmets during sports or industrial work.

Treatment

Anti-epileptic drugs (AEDs) are the main treatment for epilepsy. The medicine doesn't cure epilepsy, but helps to stop or reduce the number of seizures.

However, during a seizure, protect the casualty from falling or try to guide them gently down the floor, move objects that might injure the person, and loosen clothing around neck to ease breathing.

Check for medication and turn the person on one side (recovery position), so that fluid can leak out of the mouth.

For a child with fever convulsions, sponge the body with lukewarm water to help cool the victim.

Do not place any object on the mouth of an epileptic casualty or try to stop them from movement.

Most seizures lasts not more than 5 minutes. However, status epilepticus lasts for more than 30 minutes.

Call for an ambulance or take to hospital if the seizure lasts for more than 5 minutes.

Seizure may lead to an altered mental status, which is the change of a person's normal awareness, showing signs of confusion, disorientation, or unresponsiveness.

After a seizure, sometimes the person may also feel ashamed. Therefore, try to keep the crowd away to give them privacy.

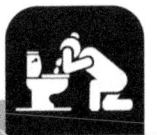

15.9 | Vomiting and Diarrhea (Cholera)

Cholera is caused by bacteria, and spreads through contaminated water or food. But flies can also spread cholera.

Symptoms are characterized by acute onset of profuse watery diarrhea ("rice-water" stools) and often vomiting.

The number of cases can rise very quickly with explosive pattern of outbreaks.

In Kenya, the national incidence of cholera has been on steady increase in recent years. In 2015, a total of 101 deaths and 4900 cases were reported.

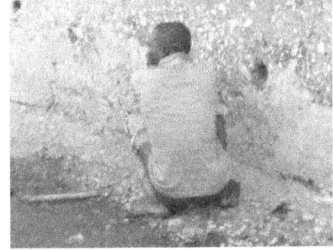

Figure 33: Cholera outbreak is the result of open defecation

Over the past, cholera has been largely confined to rural areas without toilets and urban slums with poor sanitation.

In these areas, people relieve themselves in the bush because most homes do not have toilets.

When it rains, the waste is swept into the river which is the main source of water for thousands in rural areas.

In urban slums, there is lack of sewer lines and inadequate latrines. Between 200–300 slum dwellers share one latrine.

Kibera slums, for instance, is popular of flying toilets, because residents defecate in polythene bugs and throw outside.

Treatment

The biggest danger of cholera, however, is the excessive loss of body water and salt during vomiting and diarrhea.

In severe cases, continuous fluid loss may quickly lead to extreme dehydration and shock that could be fatal.

Prompt replacement of fluid lost is the mainstay of treatment of cholera.

For mild or moderate dehydration, fluid replacement can be achieved by drinking oral rehydration solution (ORS) available in most chemists.

Locally, rehydration solution can be made by mixing 8 teaspoons of sugar and half a spoon of salt in a liter of clean water. Plenty of clean water is also fine.

However, very severely dehydrated patients, with uncontrollable vomiting or extreme fatigue that prevents drinking, should be rushed to the hospital as fast as possible for intravenous rehydration.

Prevention

Prevention is always better than cure!

Since untreated stools from cholera patients are the primary source of contamination, proper disposal of liquid waste should be undertaken to prevent contamination and secondary spread of infection.

Other prevention measures include:

- Drinking safe water, boiled or purified using chlorine tablets.

- Washing hands often with soap and safe water.

- Using latrines or burying feces.

- Cooking food well and keeping it covered.

Control

Cholera is potentially fatal if not properly managed and controlled.

To minimize the risk of cholera infection, the following measures are recommended:

- Early reporting and surveillance of cholera cases to facilitate investigation and outbreak detection.

- Environmental disinfection to prevent secondary spread in the community.

- High standard of food safety and hygiene practices.

ENVIRONMENTAL EMERGENCIES

Our bodies are designed to adjust to keep temperature within a safe range by making and getting rid of heat.

When you are too hot, the blood vessels in your skin widen to carry the excess heat to your skin's surface. You may start to sweat. As the sweat evaporates, it helps cool your body.

When you are too cold, your blood vessels narrow. This reduces blood flow to your skin to save body heat. You may start to shiver. When the muscles tremble this way, it helps to make more heat.

However, if the body becomes overwhelmed, heat and cold related emergencies can happen.

Dehydration is one major factor that contributes to heat and cold related emergencies.

Other heat related illnesses include heat cramps, heat exhaustion and heat stroke.

However, high body temperature may be as a result of fever, which is the body's normal reaction to infection.

Cold-related emergencies include frostbite and hypothermia, which can happen to anyone exposed to cold temperatures for too long, and they can be life threatening.

Children are more vulnerable to heat and cold emergencies as they adjust more slowly than adults do to changes in environmental.

They often do not think to rest when having fun and may not drink enough fluids when playing, exercising, or participating in sports.

Most people think of 'normal' body temperature as 37C. Yet, the concept of there being a normal body temperature is somewhat misleading.

The fact is, normal body temperature can vary in ranges between 36.1C to 37.2C according to a wide range of factors including a person's age, the time of day and whether someone is active or not.

Heat and cold emergencies can be prevented by following commonsense guidelines, and taking steps in extreme temperatures to maintain a normal body temperature.

Recognizing early symptoms is important to keep these conditions from worsening.

When heat or cold emergencies do occur, act quickly to get medical attention before the emergency become life-threatening.

Hyperthermia occurs when body produces more heat than it loses through radiation, convection, conduction, evaporation, and breathing.

Elderlies have higher risk for heat emergencies due to lack of mobility, impaired ability to regulate body temperature, impaired sense of thirst, and medications.

Newborns and infants are at higher risk of heat emergencies due to their impaired ability to regulate body temperature and inability to remove their own clothing.

The three main types of heat emergencies include heat cramps, heat exhaustion, and heat stroke.

Preventing Heat Emergencies

In hot environments wear lightweight clothing, rest on shades, drink adequate fluids, but avoid stimulants.

When new to a hot area, take up to 10 days to gradually acclimatize to heat and humidity before engaging in strenuous activity.

Do not leave children alone in a car, they may lock themselves inside and play with vehicles air conditioning system.

Dehydration

Dehydration is when somebody loses too much water and salt. It is dangerous and can cause death.

Vomiting, diarrhea and sweating can cause dehydration.

Dehydrated person feels thirsty, tired, and have sunken eyes. In babies, fontanel (soft spot on skull) may go down.

Give plenty of water or sugar-salt solution to a dehydrated person, by mixing 8 teaspoons of sugar, half teaspoon of salt in 1 liter of clean water.

Heat Cramps

Activity in hot environment may cause painful cramps in muscles, often on lower legs and abdominal muscles.

Signs of heat cramps include muscle pain, cramping, spasm, and heavy sweating.

Have the person stop activity and seat in a cool place, give a sports drink or water. Avoid strenuous activity for hours to avoid progression.

For abdominal cramp, continue resting in comfortable position. For leg cramps, stretch the muscle by extending the leg and flexing the ankle. Apply pressure to the crumpled area.

Seek medical attention for victims with a heart problem.

Heat Exhaustion

Activity in hot environment usually causes heavy sweating which may lead to dehydration and depletion of salt and electrolytes in the body if the person does not get enough fluids.

A victim of heat exhaustion feels thirsty, fainting, and sweats heavily, with body temperature above 38°C, but symptoms improve with moving to cool environment, removal of excess clothing, drinking water, raising legs, and rest.

You can also cool the victim by putting wet cloth on forehead, sponging skin with cool water, or spraying with water and fanning the area.

Seek medical attention if the victims condition does not improve within 30 minutes, has a heart condition or high blood pressure.

Heat exhaustion may progress to heat stroke if not treated.

Heat Stroke

Heat stroke is the most severe of heat related emergencies. It occurs when the body can no longer regulate its temperature.

Firefighters and athletes who wear heavy clothing and perform strenuous activity for long periods in hot environments are at risk for heat stroke.

A victim of heat stroke has very high body temperature, above 39°C, and an altered mental status. Other signs include seizure, nausea and head ache.

You must act quickly to lower the body temperature of heat stroke victim to increase their chances of survival.

Call for an ambulance, move victim to cool place, remove outer clothing, and cool the victim with any means such as wrapping in wet sheet, sponging with cold water, putting ice packs on the neck, armpit and groin area.

Do not give pain relievers to a heat stroke victim. If nauseating, do not give liquids.

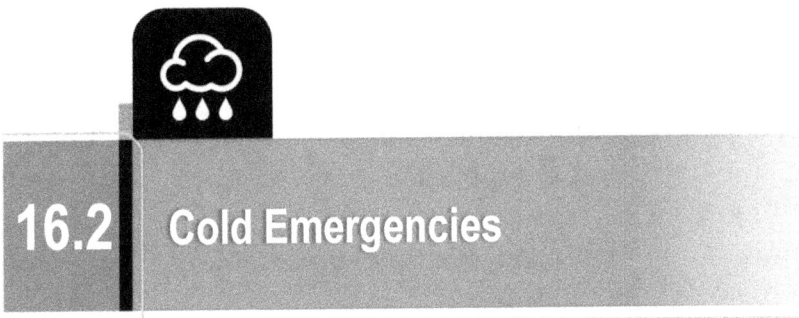

16.2 Cold Emergencies

Exposure to cold temperatures can cause either localized cold injury (frost bite) or lowering of the whole body temperature (hypothermia).

Prevention of Cold Emergencies

When planning to be outdoors for a long time, check weather forecasting, carry extra clothing, have high energy food bars like chocolate, and do not consume alcohol.

Wear a hat. Up to 50% of body heat is lost from the head.

Hypothermia

Hypothermia occurs when the body loses more heat than it produces, usually below 35 Degree Celsius.

Hypothermia occurs more easily on elderlies, people under influence of alcohol, and victims of immersion in cold water.

Young children are unable to protect themselves from cold because they have less body insulation fat, high surface area to volume ration, and they cannot shiver.

Causes of hypothermia include long exposure to cold, immersion in water, alcohol intake, or medical condition.

Signs of hypothermia include shivering, difficulty talking or moving, altered mental status, confusion, and pale, cool skin.

First aid for hypothermia include getting the victim out of the cold, removing wet clothing, and covering them with warm clothing. You can also give warm (not hot) drinks to an alert victims, but not stimulants (alcohol or caffeine).

Do not immerse victims of hypothermia in hot water or use direct heat such as hot water bottle, because rapid warming can cause heart problems.

Local Cold Injury (Frostbite)

Blood is always forced away from arms and legs to the body core when body is exposed to cold causing tissue damage.

Frostbite is the damage to tissues of a body part when exposed to prolonged cold, usually below 32 °C. Ice crystals stats to form within the cells, which damages them.

Feeling of 'pins and needles,' numbness, and lack of pain are sure signs of frostbite. Others include waxy, blue skin.

Move victim to warm environment, remove tight clothing or jewelry, warm area with warm water (37 °C - 40°C) or your groin or armpits, apply light dressing between the toes or fingers, raise affected part above heart level to reduce swelling, and seek medical attention immediately.

The victim may choose to take aspirin for pain, and drink warm liquid, but not stimulants such as alcohol.

Avoid breaking blisters, rubbing affected area, and allowing victim to walk on affected leg.

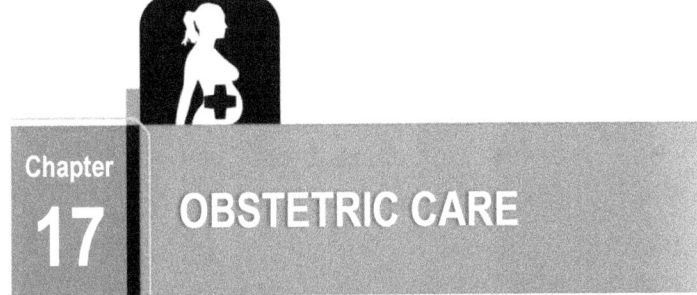

Chapter 17 — OBSTETRIC CARE

The safest place for the mother who is about to deliver her baby is in the maternity department.

At times, this is not possible and pre-hospital delivery of the baby is neccssary.

The following three cases, are some of the instances in which you should not try to transport the mother to a hospital:

- ➲ When you have no transportation available.
- ➲ When the delivery of the baby can be expected within five minutes.
- ➲ When the hospital or doctor cannot be reached, may be due to a disaster.

Even so, childbirth is a natural process, and most deliveries occur without complications.

When birth is imminent and medical help is unavailable, it is important to understand the normal course of labor and childbirth.

The mother and anyone who is helping can make the birth easier and safer by knowing exactly what is happening and how best to help.

This process of childbirth is open to infection. It is therefore imperative that you take all possible precautions against infection from yourself and from the surroundings. Ensure that you wear gloves (if available) during the process.

To avoid birth complications, it is also important for pregnant women to avoid stimulants, and consult a doctor before taking any medication or herbal supplement.

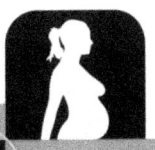

17.1 | Stages of Pregnancy

Pregnancy lasts about 40 weeks, counting from the first day of the last normal period. The weeks are grouped into three trimesters as detailed below:

First Trimester of Pregnancy (1-3 months)

During this period, mother stops menstruating, breasts become swollen, urinates more frequently, and sleeps more than usual.

During first week after conception, the mother's body produce more blood, and heart rate increases to pump extra blood.

The arms, legs, heart, lungs, and brain begins to form and fetus is 3 inches long.

Nausea and vomiting (usually called morning sickness) are worst during the second month.

Second Trimester (4-6 months)

Signs of pregnancy become more obvious with enlarged abdomen as fetus is about 13 inches.

Mother may walk and move differently due to changes in center of gravity. Fetus's fingers, toes, eyelashes and eyebrows are formed.

Third Trimester (7-9 months)

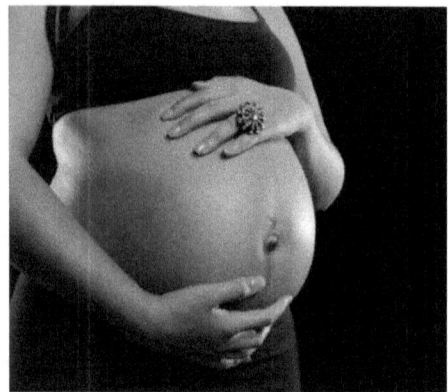

Mother may complain of backache due to muscle strain. Stretch marks may appear.

Mother urinates frequently, because the weight of the uterus presses on the bladder. She may have shortness of breath as uterus expands beneath diaphragm.

Fetus continue to grow rapidly, gaining a half pound a week and reaching a length of about 20 inches.

Fetal movement occurs often and stronger. Normally, the head of the fetus settles into the pelvis in preparation for delivery.

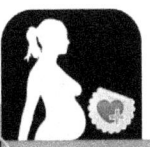

17.2 Medical Considerations for Pregnant Women

⊃ Pregnant women should lie on their left, not back, to reduce fetus pressure on abdominal blood vessels. When placed on her back, the weight of the fetus compresses major blood vessels in the abdomen, reducing amount of blood returning to the heart.

⊃ During pregnancy, a woman's center of gravity shifts and her pelvic ligaments loosen, which increases her risk for falls and injury.

⊃ The likelihood of fetal death is high, even in low electrical current, because fetus is floating on amniotic fluid with low current resistance.

⊃ Pregnant women's breathing rate is slightly faster, and blood pressure slightly lower than normal until third trimester.

⊃ The well-being of the fetus is entirely dependent on the well-being of the mother.

⊃ When giving first aid care, consider the possibility of pregnancy in any woman of childbearing age.

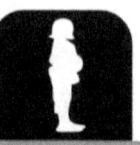

17.3 Pre-delivery Considerations

Labor with the first pregnancy is usually longer than that of subsequent deliveries.

Knowing the due date will help you know if the baby is premature or full term.

Fetus usually needs to be delivered within 18-24 hours after the bag of waters has broken.

Discharge of mucus mixed with blood is a sign that labor has begun.

The urge to push as the baby moves down the birth canal is a symptom that delivery will occur soon.

The baby's breathing may be very slow at delivery if the mother used narcotics within four hours of delivery.

Delivery is expected in a few minutes if a woman feels urge to push, crowning is present, contractions are regular lasting 45-60 seconds over a period of 1-2 minutes.

Consider delivering at scene if delivery is expected in minutes, no suitable transportation is available, or the hospital cannot be reached due to heavy traffic.

Even though you may be nervous about helping with delivery, it is important that you appear calm and confident.

Keep in mind that the mother is doing all the work. Your job is to help the mother and the new born.

Although some women have labor with relatively little pain, most women experience considerable pain that worsens as labor progresses.

If a delivering woman is irritable, and halts obscenities to you, do not take any comments she makes personally.

Always use protection like gloves, musk, and eye protection from blood and amniotic fluids which may splash.

You may need a readymade childbirth delivery kit containing scissors, thin strings, clean towel, sterile glove, sanitary pads, baby blanket, bulb syringe, and plastic bag.

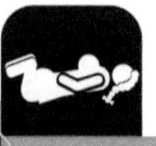

17.4 Signs and Stages of Labor

Giving birth is different for every woman, but the main sign of labour is strong, regular contractions. Other signs are breaking of waters, backache, and an urge to go to the toilet caused by the baby's head pressing on bowel.

Some women have false labor pain about 2-4 weeks before delivery, but at times it's difficult to tell the difference between false and true labor. The false labor helps to prepare a woman's body for delivery by softening the cervix.

There are three stages to labour, with the first stage being contractions that make the cervix to gradually open up.

The second stage of labour is when the cervix is fully open, and the baby moves through the vagina as the mother pushes.

The third stage is after the birth of the baby, when the womb contracts and causes placenta to come out through the vagina.

First Stage - Contractions and Opening of Womb

This stage begins with womb contractions, lasting for 30-60 seconds and occur after every 5-15 minutes. It ends with opening of the cervix.

During contraction, the womb (uterus) gets tight and then relaxes. The contractions are pushing the baby down and opening the cervix ready for the baby to go through.

In a woman who has previously not given birth, this stage lasts about 8-16 hours, and lasts 6-8 hours in a woman who have previously given birth.

Place fingers of one hand high on the uterus to feel if the abdomen become hard, indicating contraction has started. When hardness is gone, contraction has ended.

Second Stage – Delivery of the Baby

This second stage of labour begins when the cervix is fully dilated and lasts until the birth of the baby.

At this stage, there are stronger contractions lasting 45-60 seconds over a period of 2-3 minutes.

Normally, the first part that comes out of the birth canal first is the head. Buttocks or feet may descend first in breech delivery.

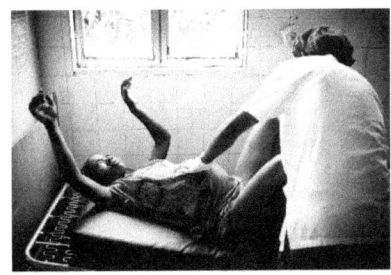

Crowning is when the presenting part remains visible from vaginal opening. This stage takes averagely 1-2 hours in a woman who has previously not given birth, and 20-30 minutes in a woman who has given birth previously.

Third Stage - Delivery of the Infant

After the baby is born, more contractions will push out the placenta.

During this process, the placenta peels from the wall of uterus exposing tiny blood vessels.

Placenta usually delivers within 15-30 minutes after infant's birth.

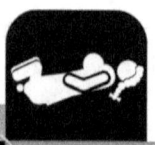

17.5 | Delivery Procedure

When the mother's cervix is completely open, she will feel an almost involuntary need to push.

When contractions begin, tell the mother to take in deep breath and hold as you count for 10 seconds, and blow it out.

Once contraction is over, the mother should begin restful breathing and relax to conserve energy for the next contraction.

Always offer words of encouragement to the mother and praise her for the progress she is making.

Delivery of the Baby

When infants head appears, cup your gloved hand over the crowning head to prevent explosive delivery.

Do not try to delay the birth by having the woman hold her legs together or any other maneuver. Do not pull out the baby's head or shoulders when coming out.

If the legs come out first and not the head, do not try to do anything. Get hospital help as quick as possible. This is a serious emergency.

If the umbilical cord is looped around the neck, gently slip it over the babies shoulder or head.

If the umbilical cord is tightly wrapped around the baby's neck, talk to the doctor, and if permitted, place two ties on the cord about 3 inches apart and cut carefully.

If there is anything covering the baby's face, gently remove it to allow the baby to breath.

Once the baby's shoulder has come out, the rest of the body will come out very quickly. Lift the baby carefully – they are slippery and can be dropped easily. Pass the baby to the mother and note the time the baby was born.

The baby may start to cry, if they do not, then check airway, breathing and flow of blood in blood vessels.

When the baby lies, make sure they lie on the side to allow mucus or fluid to drain from the mouth or nose.

Quickly dry the baby to remove blood and amniotic fluid and wrap in clean warm blanket to prevent heat loss, keeping the face exposed. Do not try to wash the infant's skin or face.

Most body heat is lost through the head. Therefore, immediately dry the baby and cover the head as soon as possible.

If the baby has not begun to breathe or is breathing very slowly, stimulate the baby by rubbing the back, chest or tapping bottom of feet.

Assess the baby's pulse by feeling the brachial pulse on the inside of the upper arm. The newborn's legs and arms are always bluish immediately after delivery, but should quickly improve if the baby is breathing normally and is kept warm.

Delivery of Umbilical Cord

When umbilical cord stops pulsating 3-5 minutes after delivery of the baby, tie a knot round the cord about a palm's length from the infant using string and a second knot at similar length and cut between the two ties using sterilized scissors.

Do not pull the umbilical cord while placenta is coming out.

The mother may continue to bleed up to a pint following delivery. Place sanitary pads, or clean cloths against the vaginal opening, but do not push.

Gently message the mother's abdomen just below the navel to help the uterus contract to stop the bleeding.

Encourage the mother to breast feed her baby. Breastfeeding stimulates the uterus to contract and decrease bleeding by constricting blood vessels.

Even with a successful delivery, the mother and infant must go to hospital because sometimes problems occur within the first 24 hours.

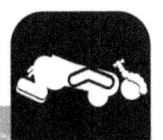

17.6   Complications of Pregnancy

Overwhelming majority of childbirth occur naturally without any complications, but you should be prepared to manage a problem if one does occur.

Pregnant women may experience complication in their pregnancy. These complications can involve the mother's health, the baby's health, or both.

Some complications are more common than others. Below are the most common pregnancy complications:

Breech Birth

Occur when infant's feet or buttocks appear first in the birth canal rather than the head.

Breech birth may cause suffocation of the infant on vaginal wall or stoppage of blood flow in the squeezed umbilical cord.

When you see a breech birth, move the woman to a kneeling position with head and chest down.

Kneeling position helps to minimize pressure on the cord and is the preferred childbirth position in breech birth situation.

You may need to open a breathing space for infant if the head does not emerge soon after the body during breech birth, but do not pull the head out.

Carefully insert one hand alongside the infants face and make a "V" with two fingers positioned on each side of the infant's nose.

Gestational Diabetes

Gestational Diabetes develops during pregnancy, when a woman's body is not making enough insulin.

Develops usually in second trimester.

Cannot be treated by pills. Most treatment is through diet or insulin.

Low Birth Weight

Caused by poor nutrition, substance use (cigarettes, alcohol, drugs).

Can be an effect of sexually transmitted disease, other contagious diseases, or no prenatal care.

When a baby is born prematurely, it stays in the hospital for up to four months.

Babies who are born at a low birth weight run the risk of respiratory infections, blindness, learning disabilities, cerebral palsy, and heart infections.

Preterm Labor

When the mother's body is trying to deliver the baby before she has reached full-term (37 weeks).

There is a risk of delivering the baby too early when the contractions are closer, stronger, and longer.

In serious situations, bed rest and medications are necessary to help the pregnancy go full-term.

Rh Negative Disease

Rh factor is determined by the presence of a protein surrounding red blood cells. Without the protein, a woman is considered Rh negative.

If the mother is Rh negative, and her child is born Rh positive, she starts to build antibodies up against the next Rh positive baby.

During the beginning of the pregnancy, the mother is tested to see if she has been sensitized. (Meaning the baby's red blood cells have been affected by the mother's developed antibodies).

RhoGAM is a hospital medication given around 28 weeks to prevent the build-up of these antibodies. RhoGAM is given again at birth, only if the baby is Rh positive.

Ectopic Pregnancy

Ectopic pregnancy occurs when a fertilized egg implants outside the womb, usually inside fallopian tube.

Initial symptoms of ectopic pregnancy include missed menstrual period, virginal bleeding over 6-8 weeks, and lower abdominal pain.

Although there are many causes of abdominal pain, you must consider lower abdominal pain in any woman of child bearing age to be due to ectopic pregnancy unless proven otherwise.

Arrange for immediate transport to closest appropriate health facility.

It's not important to determine the cause of vaginal bleeding. But what's important is to recognize that the patient needs immediate transport to hospital.

Other child birth problems include protruding cord through birth canal before childbirth (prolapsed cord), cord around neck, and bleeding after delivery.

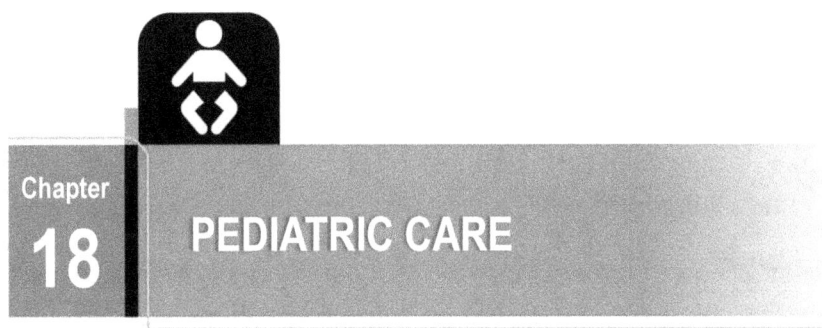

PEDIATRIC CARE

Children differ from adults anatomically, socially and in their reasoning.

When involved in the same kind of accident as adults, children may suffer quite different injuries because of their different size and anatomy.

For instance, a small child hit by a car will often sustain abdominal injuries, while adults are more likely to fracture the long bones of the legs because of their greater height.

Blunt trauma may result in bone fractures in the adult population, while the cartilaginous nature of children's bones tends to prevent them from fracturing.

The things children do and their changing levels of maturity predispose them to different patterns of injury from adults.

Children are less likely to be involved in motor vehicle accidents or industrial accidents than their parents.

Instead, they fall from playground equipment, and are generally at risk in proportion to their level of reasoning and social development.

Adolescents consciously engage in risk-taking behaviors, while toddlers do not have the information or judgement to recognize and avoid imminent danger.

Protective equipment and clothing is more problematic for children than adults.

The varying and constantly changing sizes of growing children make correct sizing of helmets or car restraints difficult and expensive for families.

Older children may succumb to peer group pressure and refuse to use protective wear such as knee splints, wrist guards and helmets.

The following sections therefore outlines these differences, and how they influence the assessment and management of childhood trauma.

18.1 Anatomical differences in children

Children and infants differ, both anatomically and physiologically, from adults.

These differences will have an impact on the assessment and management of pediatric trauma or illness.

However it is important to recognize that the basic principles of trauma care - airway, breathing and circulation - remain the same, regardless of the age of the patient.

When involved in the same kind of accident as adults, children may suffer quite different injuries because of their different size and anatomy.

For instance, blunt trauma may result in bone fractures in adults, while the cartilaginous nature of children's bones tends to prevent them from fracturing.

The following are some of the bodily differences:

- *Smaller airway*, therefore, greater risk of chocking and airway obstruction from small foreign bodies.

- *Tongue is large in proportion to the mouth* means that, in the child, the tongue is more likely to obstruct the airway than in the adult.

- *A child's head is proportionately larger and heavier than an adults is until about four years of age*, hence they flex their heads forward when placed on a flat surface. To achieve a neutral position in cervical spine immobilization, it may be necessary to place a pad under the trunk of the infant.

- *Breathe exclusively through the nose* in the first 4-6 months of age, and will experience respiratory distress if the nose is blocked.

- *Cartilaginous airway* makes it more subject to collapse and obstruction than the adult airway if the child is not positioned appropriately.

- *Breathe using diaphragm than chest muscles.* This means that with inspiration the ribs only move up, and not up-and-out, like the adult rib cage.

- *Significantly higher metabolic rates than adults*, and therefore have a higher oxygen demand, which in turn results in higher respiratory rates. The amount of oxygen a child requires is about twice that of an adolescent or an adult.

- *Blood volume is relatively larger, but absolute volume is smaller*, hence bleeding can be life-threatening.

- *Bulging fontanel* suggest a rise in intracranial pressure, which may be a result of intracranial bleeding.

- *Thinner cranial bones* of children do not afford as much protection to the brain tissue as the thicker bones of the adult skull.

- *Relatively larger size of the head* results in a higher center of gravity, which in turn contributes to a higher incidence of head trauma in children.

- *Relatively small size*, hence greater likelihood that a single impact will injure multiple organ systems.

- *The larger surface-area to body-mass ratio* results in greater heat loss for infants and children.

- *Infants have poorly developed temperature-regulating mechanisms,* such as shivering, sweating, and movement.

18.1 Developmental Stages of Children

From helpless newborn to active teenage, babies grow and change at an astounding pace, and every month brings new and exciting developments.

These new developments present unique functions in the children's body that need to be considered when providing care, as highlighted in the subsequent sections.

Infants (below one year)

Infants are completely dependent on others for their needs.

When they cry, it is an indication of pain, hunger, extreme temperature or dirty diaper.

Avoid loud noises, bright light, and quick, jerky movements. Instead, use calm, soothing voice, and handle infants gently but firmly.

Infants must be kept warm and covered as much as possible, particularly the head, which is the largest surface area.

The risk of choking begins at approximately six months of age. Be careful not to leave small objects within an infant's reach.

Never shake or jiggle an infant or child. It can lead to severe brain damage or death.

Toddlers (1-3 years)

A toddler is always on the move. As a result, they are prone to injuries.

Toddlers view illness and injury as punishment.

Most toddlers experience strong anxiety when separated from their mothers or caregivers.

A toddler is more cooperative if given comfort objects such as blanket, stuffed animals, or toy.

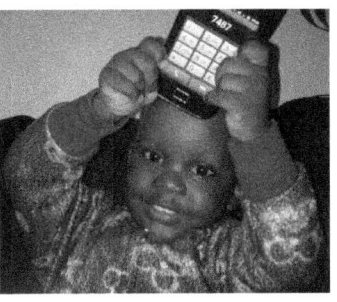

Toddlers are distrustful of strangers, and may scream, cry or kick to resist examination or treatment by strangers.

Encourage a child's trust by talking to, and gaining cooperation of the caregiver first, to make them more at ease.

Approach a child slowly and talk to her at eye level, using simple words and short phrases with calm, reassuring tone of voice.

Although a child may not understand your words, they will respond to your tone.

Assess a child from feet moving upward to head. If possible, ask caregiver to remove clothing.

Preschoolers (4-5 years)

Preschoolers are afraid of the unknown, the dark, being left alone, and adults who look or act mean. They are highly imaginative and may think their illness or injury is punishment for bad behavior or thoughts.

Assess and treat preschooler child in upright position if possible. They may feel vulnerable and out of control when lying down.

Tell the child what to be done and how it will feel as they are always curious such as pain.

Use understandable words when talking to children e.g. "am going to see how fast your heart is beating," instead of "checking your pulse."

Children are self-centered – they imagine the world revolves around them. Paying attention to their world improves your ability to assess and care for them.

School age children (6-12 years)

School-age children are less dependent on their caregivers and cooperative than are younger children. They fear pain, permanent injury and are afraid of blood and prolonged separation from their caregivers.

They are modest and does not like their body exposed to strangers.

Talk to the child directly about what happened, even if you obtained history from the caregiver.

Explain procedures, choosing your words carefully e.g. the phrase "I am taking your pulse" will make him wonder why you are taking it away and when he will get it back.

Honesty is very important. If you're going to do something that causes pain, warn the child just before the procedure so that he does not have long time to think about it.

Do not threaten the child if he is uncooperative.

Adolescents (13-18 years)

Adolescents often show inconsistent and unpredictable behavior, but prefer to be treated as adults.

Expect an adolescent to have so many questions about your actions and their conditions.

Do not bargain with an adolescent in order to do what you need to do.

Recognize the tendency of adolescents to overreact, and do not become angry with an emotional and hysterical adolescent.

Adolescents fear pain, permanent damage, and change in appearance or death. They may go back and forth between modesty and open displays of their bodies.

Some adolescents may prefer to be assessed privately, away from their parents and caregivers.

Peers are a major influence in the life of an adolescent. When providing care, an adolescent may prefer to have a peer close by for reassurance.

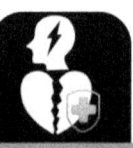

I n disasters, for every one physical injury, there may be 4-5 psychological injuries.

People may feel dazed or even numb after surviving a disaster. They may also feel sad, helpless, or anxious. In spite of the tragedy, some people just feel happy to be alive.

It is not unusual to have bad memories or dreams. You may avoid places or people that remind you of the disaster.

You might have trouble sleeping, eating, or paying attention. Many people have short tempers and get angry easily. These are all normal reactions to stress.

Sometimes the stress can be too much to handle alone, and have long-term problems, including:

- ⮑ Post-traumatic stress disorder

- ⮑ Depression

- ⮑ Self-blame

- ⮑ Suicidal thoughts

- ⮑ Alcohol or drug abuse

If your emotional reactions are getting in the way of your relationships, work, or other important activities, talk to a counselor or your doctor. Treatments are available.

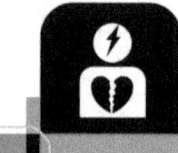

19.1 Psychological Disorders

Psychological disorders, also known as mental disorders, are behavioral patterns that are unacceptable to the victim, family, or community.

The disorders can be due to situational stressors such as disasters, death, or failed relationship.

It can also be due to illness such as poisoning, seizure, low blood sugar or head trauma.

Psychiatric conditions such as panic, bizarre thinking, and use of stimulants may also cause psychological disorders.

Some of the mental disorders are highlighted below:

Altered Mental Status

Reduced oxygenated blood supply to the brain may cause altered responsiveness. Other causes include low blood sugar, panic, head injuries and illness.

The appropriate first aid for altered mental status is to care for the underlying causes of the altered status.

While giving care, protect yourself from casualty with altered mental status, as they often behave irrationally with extreme strength.

Take steps to calm and reassure the victim, following these guidelines:

- ⮑ Stay at a safe distance away from the victim until your help is accepted.

- ⮑ Move calmly and slowly, touching the victim only when necessary.

- ⮑ Ask for the victim's name, and use it when speaking. Make eye contact, and stay at the victim's eye level.

- ⮑ Speak in caring, reassuring voice, but do not give false assurances.

- ⮑ Avoid being judgmental, and do not assume the victim is intoxicated with drugs.

- ⮑ Do not argue with the victim. Instead, let the victim know you understand their concerns.

Anxiety and Panic

Anxiety is the state of worry and agitation that is usually triggered by a vague or imagined situation, while panic attack is an intense fear that occurs for no apparent reason, with symptoms such as sweating or trembling.

A little anxiety is good to the point it increase desire to perform, however, it may increase to a level that interferes with thinking and problem-solving.

Anxiety normally goes away after a stressful situation that caused it is over. But anxiety disorder lasts for months.

While it is normal to fear, some people are prone to extreme anxiety and may have panic attack.

Always be composed and gentle when calming and reassuring a casualty with signs of panic and anxiety.

Phobia

Phobia is an irrational constant fear of a specific activity, object or situation. A phobic reaction resembles panic attack.

Some phobias are common and usually do not create a problem because the person simply avoids the activity, object, or situation.

Depression

Someone with a depression often feels sad, worthless, discouraged and may experience weight loss, diarrhea, difficulty sleeping, appetite loss, and thoughts of suicide.

It is important to make attempts to communicate with a victim who seems depressed. Follow these guidelines:

- Encourage the victim to talk, acknowledging that the victim seems sad and ask why.

- Be reassuring and empathetic, providing comforts to make the victim open up.

- If the victim is crying, do not stop them.

- If the victim complains about something, do not give false reassurance, but offer alternatives for help.

- Be alert for possibility of suicide.

Bipolar Disorder

A person with bipolar disorder has alternating episodes of mood elevation and disorder.

Paranoia

Paranoia is a mental disorder characterized by excessive suspiciousness, and false beliefs that the victim believes are true, despite facts to the contrary.

Paranoid casualty believe that people are following, harassing them, or reading their minds. They carry grudges, recalling wrongs done to them years earlier.

Suicidal feelings

Most people who commit suicide express their intention beforehand. Follow these guidelines if you are caring for a person who may be suicidal:

- Take the person seriously and listen to what they are saying. Talk calmly and supportively.

- Do not argue the person out of committing suicide, but let them know you understand and care.

- Involve friends and family if possible.

- Do not leave the person alone unless your own safety is threatened.

- Do not let the person drive, and remove any weapon or drugs that might be used in suicide attempt.

19.2   Grieving Process

G rief is a normal response that helps people cope with the loss of someone or something that had a great meaning to them.

It is a very personal process where a person may pass through five stages including denial, anger, bargaining, depression and acceptance.

Denial (Not me)

During this stage a person is unable or refuses to accept what has happened.

Common reaction in this state include 'this can't be happening.'

When dealing with a casualty at this stage, try to find information from close friend or family.

Anger (Why me?)

A person's anger may be related to discomfort, limitation of activity or inability to control the situation.

The person can be abusive, irritable, and often experiences guilt and blames with common reactions such as 'if only I had....', ' why is this happening to me.'

When dealing with an angry person, remember that your safety is your priority and do not take insults personally.

It is not necessary to agree with the person, but do not challenge how he is feeling. In addressing anger, you can:

- Be empathetic and talk to him in calm, controlled tone.

- Discuss how the anger is affecting their life (e.g. relationship with family and friends).

- Normalize the experience of anger, by discussing how anger can increase conflict and push others away.

- Ask the person to identify changes that they would like to make to address their anger.

- Compare how holding on to the anger versus letting go of anger can help or hurt them.

- Emphasize that some anger is normal and helpful, while too much anger can undermine them a lot.

Some anger management skills that you can suggest include:

- Take a "time out" or "cool down" (walk away and calm down, do something else for a while).

- Blow off steam through physical exercise e.g. pushups.

- Remind yourself that anger will not help you achieve what you want, and may harm relationships.

- Distract yourself with positive activities like listening to upbeat music or going to religious services.

- Look at your situation from another's viewpoint, or find reasons your anger may be over the top.

⊃ For parents, have another family member or friend temporarily supervise your children's activities while you are feeling particularly angry or irritable.

Bargaining (okay, but first let me...)

The person is willing to do anything to change what is happening. He bargains with himself, family, God or medics.

Bargaining reflects the persons need for time to accept the situation.

Depression (I don't care of anything)

A depressed person is usually sad, silent, withdrawn, experience difficulty concentrating, and rejects help.

Be supportive and nonjudgmental whenever care is needed.

Acceptance (okay I am not afraid)

The person has come to terms with his loss or change of circumstances and is learning to live with it. He may not be happy, but believes he has done everything possible.

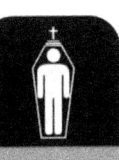

Acute grief reactions are likely to be intense and prevalent among those who have suffered the death of a loved one or close friend.

They may feel sadness over the death, guilt over not having been able to prevent the death, and wishing for reunion (including dreams of seeing the person again).

Although painful to experience at first, these grief reactions are healthy responses that reflect the significance of the death.

Over time, grief reactions tend to include more pleasant thoughts and activities, such as telling positive stories about a loved one, and comforting ways to remember them.

When a survivor does want to talk with you about the loved one, you should listen quietly, and not feel compelled to talk a lot. Do not probe.

Care for Bereaved Adults

Some of the things you can do include:

- Reassure grieving individuals that what they are experiencing is understandable.

- Use the deceased person's name, rather than referring to them as "the deceased."

➲ Tell them that if they continue to experience feelings of grief or depression, talking to a member of the clergy or to a counselor is advisable.

Don't say things such as:

➲ I know how you feel.

➲ It was probably for the best.

➲ He is better off now.

➲ It was her time to go.

➲ You should be glad he passed quickly.

➲ Let's talk about something else.

➲ That which doesn't kill us makes us stronger.

➲ You did everything you could.

➲ It's good that you are alive.

➲ It's good that no one else died.

➲ It could be worse; you still have a brother.

➲ Everything happens for the best.

➲ (To a child) You are the man of the house now.

If the grieving person says any of the above things, you can respectfully acknowledge the feeling or thought, but don't initiate a statement like these yourself.

Child and adolescent understanding of death varies depending on age, prior experience, and cultural values.

- Pre-school children may not understand that death is permanent, and may believe that if they wish it, the person can return. They need help to confirm the physical reality of a person's death. They may be concerned about something bad happening to another family member.

- School-age children may understand the physical reality of death, but may personify death as a monster. In longing for their return, they may experience upsetting feelings of the "ghostlike" presence of the lost person, but not tell anyone.

- Adolescents generally understand that death is irreversible. Losing a family member or friend can trigger rage and impulsive decisions, such as quitting school, running away, or abusing substances. These issues need prompt attention by the family or school.

It can be helpful for a child to attend a funeral. Although emotionally challenging, funerals help children accept the physical reality of the death, that is part of grieving.

If not included, children can feel left out of something important to the family.

Parents/caregivers should give children a choice whether or not to attend a funeral or other ritual. They may be encouraged, but should not be pressured.

Attending to Spiritual Issues

It is common for people to rely on religious and spiritual beliefs as a way to cope with the death of a loved one.

Survivors may use religious language to talk about what is happening or want to engage in prayer or other religious practices.

In order to assist survivors with spiritual needs after a death, obtain contact and establish linkage with the local religious group.

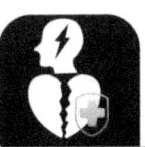

These core actions of providing early assistance need to be addressed in a flexible way, using strategies that meet the specific needs of children, families and adults.

The amount of time spent on each action varies from person to person, and with different circumstances according to need.

Contact and Engagement

The first contact with a survivor is important. It establishes an effective helping relationship and increases the victim's receptiveness to further help.

- Politely observe first, don't intrude. Then ask simple respectful questions to determine how you may help.

- Introduce yourself with your name and role.

- Often, the best way to make contact is to provide relief assistance (food, water, blankets).

- Ask for permission to talk to the victim, and explain that you are there to see if you can be of help.

- Invite the person to sit, ensure privacy, and give the person your full attention.

- Speak calmly and refrain from looking around or being distracted.

- Find out whether there is any pressing problem that needs immediate attention, such as medical concerns.

- When making contact with children, first make a connection and get permission of the parent.

- If you speak with a child in distress when no adult is present, find a parent or caregiver as soon as possible.

- Maintain the highest level of confidentiality possible in any conversation you have with survivors.

For example, in making initial contact, you might say:

Adult/ Caregiver	Hello. My name is _____. I work with _____. I'm checking in with people to see how they are doing, and to see if I can help in any way. Is it okay if I talk to you for a few minutes? May I know your name? Thank you Mrs. Marwa, before we talk, is there something right now that you need, like some water or fruit juice?
Adolescent/ Child	And is this your daughter? (Get on child's eye level, smile and greet the child, using their name and speaking softly.) Hi Lisa, I'm _____ and I'm here to try to help you and your family. Is there anything you need right now? There is some water and juice over there, and we have a few toys in those boxes.

Safety and Comfort

Promoting safety and comfort can reduce distress and worry.

Comfort and safety can be supported in a number of ways, including helping survivors:

- Do things that are active (rather than passive waiting), practical, and familiar.

- For children, toys they can hold and take care of can help them to soothe themselves.

- Get current accurate information, while avoiding exposure to inaccurate or upsetting information.

- Get connected with available resources for help.

- Get information about how responders are making the situation safer.

- Get connected with others who have shared similar experiences.

- Contact relatives, if they are available, to further insure safety, nutrition, medication and rest.

- Facilitate group and social interactions with people who are coping adequately with the situation.

- Avoid being near others who appear very agitated and emotionally overwhelmed.

- If survivors have been exposed to rumors, help to clarify and correct misinformation.

- Helping children reconnect quickly with their caregivers.

- For unaccompanied child, ask for their name, parents and siblings names, or school, and notify authorities.

- Protect survivors from exposure to additional trauma reminders, such as sights, sounds, or smells.

- Protect survivors from excessive viewing of media coverage. It can be highly upsetting, especially for children.

Stabilization

Expression of strong emotions, numbing, and anxiety are normal and healthy responses to traumatic stress, and may not require stabilization.

However, extremely high arousal, numbing, or extreme anxiety can interfere with sleep, eating, decision-making, parenting, and other life tasks.

The following steps will help to stabilize the majority of distressed individuals:

- Respect the person's privacy, and give them a few minutes before you intervene.

- Remain calm and present, rather than talk to the person, as this may contribute to emotional overload.

- Stand close by doing other tasks while being available should the person need or wish to receive help.

- Offer support and help them focus on specific manageable feelings, thoughts, and goals.

- Give information that orients them to the surroundings, such as steps they may consider.

A technique called "grounding" may be helpful. It works by turning attention from internal thoughts back to the outside world.

Here are the steps:

Step 1: Sit in a comfortable position with your legs and arms uncrossed.

Step 2: Breathe in and out slowly and deeply.

Step 3: Look around you and name five non-distressing objects that you can see.

Step 4: Breathe in and out slowly and deeply.

Step 5: Next, name five non-distressing sounds you can hear.

Step 6: Breathe in and out slowly and deeply.

Step 7: Next, name five non-distressing things you can feel.

Step 8: Breathe in and out slowly and deeply.

Information Gathering

Gathering and clarifying information begins immediately after contact, and is ongoing throughout the session.

As immediate needs and concerns are identified and addressed, it is useful to gather and clarify additional information.

Adapt interventions for specific individuals, and prioritize your interventions to meet these needs.

It may be especially useful for the provider to ask some questions to clarify the following:

- Nature and severity of disaster experiences, as well as concerns about ongoing threat.

- Death of a family member or close friend.

- Separations or safety of loved ones.

- Physical illness and need for medications.

- Losses incurred as a result of the disaster (home, business, or personal property).

- Thoughts about causing harm to self or others.

- Lack of adequate supportive social network.

- Prior alcohol or drug use.

- Prior exposure to trauma or psychological problems.

- Specific concerns of interference with anticipated developmental activities.

Relief Assistance

Ongoing harsh conditions and continuing problems resulting from a disaster can add significantly to the stress level of the survivor.

Providing people with needed resources such as food, clothing and shelter increases hope and restore dignity:

- Identify the most immediate need.

- Talk with the survivor to clarify the need.

- Discuss an action plan and address the need.

Connection with Social Supports

Help victims to establish contacts with primary support persons, including family members, friends, and community helping resources.

Social support include:

- Emotional Support: hugs, a listening ear, understanding, love, acceptance.

- Social Connection: feeling like you fit in and have things in common with other people.

- Feeling Needed: feeling that people appreciate you, that you are valued, useful and productive.

- Reassurance: having people help you have confidence in yourself and your abilities to face challenges.

- Reliable Support: having people who will be there for you in case you need them.

- Advice and Information: showing you how to do something or cope in positive ways.

- Physical Assistance: helping you do things, like fixing up your house, and helping you do paperwork.

- Material Assistance: getting things like food, clothing, shelter, medicine, building materials or money.

Coping with Traumatic Event

There are a number of steps you can take to build emotional well-being and gain a sense of control following a disaster.

Such coping methods that are likely to be helpful include:

- Give yourself time to adjust and anticipate that this will be a difficult time in your life.

- Ask for support from people who care about you and who will listen and empathize with your situation.

- Communicate your experience and express what you are feeling in whatever ways you feel comfortable.

- Spending time with others to help you realize that you are not alone in your reactions and emotions.

- Participating in a support group.

- Avoid alcohol and drugs because they can be a numbing diversion that could delay active coping.

- Avoid making major life decisions like switching jobs.

- Get adequate rest, nutrition, exercise.

- Engage in positive distracting activities, such as sports.

- Try to maintain a normal schedule if possible.

- Using calming self-talk.

- Using relaxation methods and breathing exercises help reduce feelings of tension.

- Seek help from licensed counsellor if you notice persistent feelings of distress or hopelessness.

Linkage with Collaborative Services

Psychological first aid is not the final care, and there is need to link survivors with licensed mental health practitioners for further professional care.

Examples of situations requiring a referral include:

- An acute medical problem that needs immediate attention.

- An acute mental health problem that needs immediate attention.

- Worsening of a pre-existing medical, emotional or behavioral problem.

- Threat of harm to self or others.

- Cases involving domestic, child, or elder abuse (be aware of reporting laws).

- When medication is needed for stabilization.

- When pastoral counseling is desired.

- Ongoing difficulties with coping (4 weeks or more after the disaster).

- When the survivor asks for a referral.

In addition, the survivors may want you to reconnect them to the first responders that provided them services in the primary stages of the disaster, including paramedics, police, firefighters, etc.

REFERENCES AND RESOURCES

Alire Camila (2000) *Library Disaster Planning and Recovery Handbook*. New York. Neal-Schuman

Barbara Aenhlert (2007) *Emergency Medical Responder. First Responder in Action*. New York. McGraw-Hill

Barbara Aenhlert (2009) *Emergency Medical Technician. EMT in Action*. New York. McGraw-Hill

Birdwood George, Eaglestone Frank, Fearnley Fred et al (1986) *Emergency. What to do in an emergency*. New York. Reader's Digest

Cote A.E. (2006) *Fire Protection Handbook*. Quincy MA. National Fire Protection

David TC(2007). *First Aid. Taking Action*. New York. McGraw-Hill

Deborah D. Halsted, Richard P. Jasper, Felicia M. Little (2005) *Disaster Planning*. New York. Neal-Schuman Publishers

Lynn RM, Marie ZC, Jeanettia MR (2005). *Health Safety and Nutrition for the Young Child. Sixth Edition*. USA. Thomson Delmar learning

Quarantelli E.L. (1983) *Delivery of emergency medical care in disasters: Assumptions and Realities*. New York. Irvington Publishers, Inc.

R. Howard and R. Sawyer (2003) *Terrorism and Counterterrorism: Understanding the New Security System*. New York. McGraw-Hill

Sheila Sorrentino (1999) *Assisting with Patient Care*. Missouri. Mosby, Inc.

Shelley E.T., Letitia A.P., David O.S. (2006) *Social Psychology*. London. Pearson Prentice Hall

U.S. Department of Homeland Security (2016), *"Incident Command System,"* www.fema..gov (accessed January 9, 2016)

Will Chapleau, Angel Clark Burba, Peter Pons, et al (2008) *The Paramedic*. New York. McGraw-Hill

www.nation.co.ke

www.standardmedia.co.ke

www.the-star.co.ke

INDEX

ABOUT THE AUTHOR

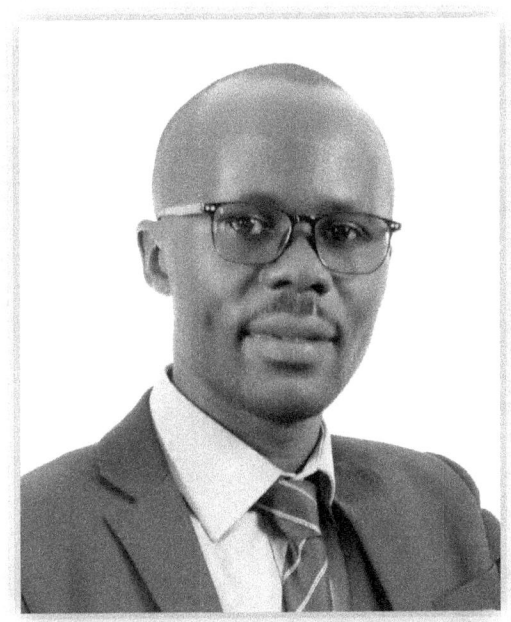

Fred Majiwa is a Disaster Expert with many years of experience as a senior manager at the St John Ambulance. Some of the epic rescue operations he has been involved include Naivasha chemical explosion accident, where 43 people lost their lives; Westgate Mall terror attack in which 67 people were shot dead; as well as numerous incidents of collapsing building and road accidents among others.

He has earned certifications in Disaster Preparedness and Emergency Operations Management. In addition, he holds a Marketing Degree and Post-Graduate Diploma in Public Relations Management.

He has been a member of several technical working groups, including the National Platform for Disaster Risk Reduction, Referral and Emergency Medical Services Policy Formulation Group, as well as Election Contingency Planning Committee among others.